Dear God,
It's Cancer

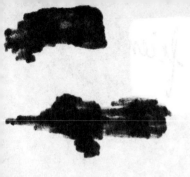

Other Books by Gerald R. McDermott

One Holy and Happy Society:
The Public Theology of Jonathan Edwards

Seeing God:
Twelve Reliable Signs of True Spirituality

Dear God, It's Cancer

A Medical and Spiritual Guide for
Patients and Their Families

**William A. Fintel, M.D.,
and Gerald R. McDermott, Ph.D.**

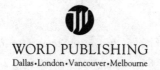

WORD PUBLISHING

Dallas・London・Vancouver・Melbourne

Unless otherwise indicated, Scripture quotations in this book
are from The Holy Bible, New International Version (NIV).
Copyright © 1973, 1978, 1984 by International Bible Society.
Used by permission of Zondervan Publishing House.
All rights reserved.

Quotations marked NJB are from The New Jerusalem Bible,
copyright © 1985 by Darton, Longman & Todd, Ltd.
and Doubleday and Company, Inc.

Quotations marked KJV are from the
King James Version of the Bible.

Quotations marked NASB are from the
New American Standard Bible © The Lockman Foundation
1960, 1962, 1963, 1968, 1971, 1972, 1973, 1975, 1977.

Quotations marked TEV are from The Good News Bible, Today's English Version.
Old Testament: Copyright © American Bible Society 1976; New Testament:
Copyright © American Bible Society 1966, 1971, 1976.

Library of Congress Cataloging-in-Publication Data
Fintel, William A.
Dear God, it's cancer : a medical and spiritual guide for patients and
their families / William A. Fintel and Gerald R. McDermott. — Rev. ed.
p.   cm.
Includes index.
ISBN 0-8499-4041-9 (trade paper)
1. Cancer—Popular Works.   2. Cancer—Religious aspects.
I. McDermott, Gerald R. (Gerald Robert)   II. Fintel, William A.
Medical and spiritual guide to living with cancer.   III. Title.
RC263.F5265   1997
616.99'4—dc21
97-11438
CIP

Printed in the United States of America

7 8 9 0 1 2   QBP   9 8 7 6 5 4 3 2 1

To John and Joan McDermott
and Norm and Jo Fintel
who gave us life and love

Contents

Foreword ix

Preface xi

Introduction: Why This Book? xv

1. What Is Cancer?
   How Good Cells Go Wrong 1

2. What Causes Cancer?
   Biological, Environmental, and Lifestyle Triggers 11

3. Has It Spread? How Far?
   Tests and Procedures You Might Expect 26

4. What Kind of Cancer Is It?
   Six Common Types of Cancer 46

5. What Can You Do for Me, Doc?
   Surgery, Radiation, Chemotherapy,
   and Biological Treatments 109

6. What Are My Rights?
   What to Expect As a Cancer Patient 129

7. How Do I Pay My Bills?
   Insurance, Medicare, and Other Strategies 137

8. What about Coffee Enemas?
   Recognizing False Promises—Medical and Spiritual 153

9. Why Me, God?
   The Age-Old Problem of Evil—And Some Answers
   We Can't Accept 175

10. Is Cancer Part of God's Plan?
Some Promising Answers to the Age-Old Question 181

11. What to Think When There Are No Answers
Coming to Terms with God's Mystery 199

12. How Do I Cope?
Sources of Spiritual Peace and Strength 204

13. Dare I Hope for Healing?
A Balanced Approach to the Possibility of Getting Well ..223

14. Why Not Suicide?
Another Look at the Kevorkian Approach 257

15. What Is Hospice?
Dying with Dignity 274

16. Is There Life after Cancer?
*How to Live Day to Day
Once Everything Has Changed* 284

Appendix: For Further Help 301

Notes 304

Glossary 315

Index 323

Foreword

One of the greatest challenges for almost all cancer patients is acquiring the knowledge they need to fully understand what a diagnosis of cancer means. Their doctors are probably giving them the life-changing and potentially life-threatening news about their diagnosis while simultaneously trying to give them a crash course in medical terminology and procedures. Whatever critical information is presented about the world of cancer they have found themselves thrust into is lost in a fog of utter shock and paralyzing numbness. The doctors might as well be talking to the wall. So home they go, often not remembering what was said except the one word that will change their lives forever: cancer.

And when the shock begins to subside, questions can totally consume their thoughts. "How did I get cancer?" "What will the treatments be like?" "Should I get a second opinion?" But now they are driving home or trying to explain to anxious family members and friends what has happened. Where can they go to ask questions? Who is awake with them at midnight when they try to make sense of the chemotherapy they start the next morning? Who will patiently sit with them while they try desperately to absorb the foreign language and culture of the medical world they will now live in. Who will repeat the same information over and over again until they not only understand it, but know what further questions to ask?

It's not that the medical profession is negligent in providing information; it's just that the individual diagnosed with cancer has a lot to learn, and fast. Few physicians have that kind of time or availability.

My wife Jan and I had been discussing the tremendous need for one great resource that could provide the valuable knowledge that the cancer patients and families we work with at our cancer ministry so desperately need. We knew from our own experience with cancer, how absolutely vital it was that we learn as much as possible as quickly as possible. But we couldn't find one book that didn't gloss over the more difficult issues (see Chapter 9, "Why Me, God?"), didn't require a medical dictionary to understand, and one that dealt not only with the physical aspects of cancer, but the emotional and spiritual aspects as well. Cancer touches every part of your life. It leaves no area unscathed. We knew this from our own experience.

William Fintel and Gerald McDermott must have had the same conversation as Jan and I. Only they had the knowledge and training to do something about it. You're holding it in your hands. And it is the answer to our prayers as well as those of countless families who find themselves searching for answers to some of the most difficult questions they have ever had to face.

For over two years we have made this book available through our ministry, Dave Dravecky's Outreach of Hope. The response we have received is overwhelming. Many patients tell us it is the most valuable resource they have been given. Many use it as a resource book, looking up the information they need, when they need it. Others read it cover to cover and then go back over the chapters that specifically pertain to them.

It has recently been updated to include four new chapters. In keeping with their straightforward approach, the authors added an especially important chapter on Physician Assisted Suicide. Their clear, well-thought-out presentation of this volatile issue is absolutely excellent and voices many of the concerns that the majority of Americans have with this alarming trend.

My only critique with Dear God, It's Cancer is that it wasn't written earlier, when I was first diagnosed.

Dave Dravecky

Preface

We're often asked where we got the idea for this book. Since we've worked so closely together on this project, we thought we'd both tell the story.

Gerry: It all started in the fall of 1990, when we first met. I was giving a series of lectures on Reformation theology at Bill's church.

Bill: I couldn't get over Gerry's ability to bring theology down to my level.

Gerry: I was impressed—and a bit put off at first!—by Bill's bold, hard-hitting questions. He kept pressing me when my answers weren't good enough for him. But I was also excited to find a layman with such keen interest in theology. So I asked him if he wanted to get together for lunch some time.

Bill: Several days later, over burgers at Mac and Bob's (a great restaurant in Salem, Virginia), I kept pushing Gerry on the relationship between our human will and God's will. We didn't get it resolved, but the discussion was fun, and I learned some more. And then it suddenly occurred to me that Gerry might be the answer to a problem.

For years I've struggled to explain the science and art of medicine in ways my cancer patients can understand. My explanations of medical terms and problems seemed to work pretty well, but I had real difficulty answering questions about faith. My crude attempts to relate God to suffering usually fell flat.

So I told Gerry how nice it would be to have a book that offered easy-to-understand answers to the toughest medical *and* spiritual questions. Such a resource would make my job as an oncologist so much easier.

Gerry: I asked Bill if there wasn't already such a book on the market.

Bill: I told him I didn't think so. On hospital nightstands I had seen books about cancer and books about God and prayer. But the books on cancer were usually too long and technical for most patients, and the books on healing and God often didn't seem believable.

Gerry: Then Bill told me nonchalantly, "Gerry, I'm neither a writer nor a theologian. But maybe you and I could work together on a book that says it all."

Bill: Gerry was the right person to present such a weighty proposition to. Before we left the restaurant, we had already sketched out an outline for twelve chapters!

That was the beginning of two years of burning the midnight oil and taxing our families' patience to complete what you have before you. Many people helped us with this book. Although we can't name all of the generous folks who lent their time and expertise, we want to give public thanks to a chosen few. Robert Benne, for instance, gave encouragement in the very first stages, when we weren't sure how to proceed, and he provided invaluable assistance throughout the project; Stephen Wike helped us make a critical connection. Luci Shaw, Philip Yancey, and Dr. Donald Bray carved time out of their hectic schedules to give deeply appreciated input at an early stage. Roland Seaboldt, our tutor for the first year, helped us shape our first draft. Laura Kendall, our editor at Word, could not have been easier to work with. And Anne Christian Buchanan, our final-version editor for the first edition, deserves a special word of thanks. Her keen insight and deft pen (or computer cursor!) have saved us much embarrassment and made this a much better book.

We also want to thank our colleagues for their professional and technical advice: Freeman Sleeper, Ph.D.; Ron Oetgen, Ph.D.; Vern Miller, Ph.D.; Alan Pieratti, Ph.D.; Paul D. Richards, M.D.; Rodney Poffenberger, M.D.; Mary Ella Zellenik, M.D.; David Randolph, M.D.; Ann Massey, M.D.; Donald "Skip" Trump, M.D.; William C. Ward, M.D.; Hal Habecker, Th.M., D.Min.; and Rev. Quigg Lawrence. We are grateful to Sherry Robertson for her word-processing help and to Jean Deel, Bill's nurse, for going beyond the call of duty. Brenda Bowers helped us more than she knows through her enthusiasm and critical insight. Joanna Benne's experienced eye helped sharpen and deepen some of the chapters. We also want to gratefully acknowledge the patients at Lewis-Gale Regional Cancer Center for their courage and faith, which have taught us much.

We thank College Lutheran Church for inviting us to do our first seminar on God and cancer. That seminar, and the congregation's critical suggestions, helped refine our thinking and encouraged us to see this project through.

Finally, a special "thank you" to Jean McDermott and Connie Fintel for exercising the patience of Job and the wisdom of Solomon in order to accommodate their scribbling husbands. And our two clans of boys—Ryan, Ross, and Sean McDermott; Andrew, Stephen, Michael, and David Fintel—deserve our appreciation for humoring their dads when they were obsessed with "the cancer book."

Gerry McDermott and Bill Fintel

Preface to the Revised Edition

It's been four years since the first edition of this book appeared under the title *Living with Cancer*. We've been gratified by the responses of readers. Most have reported enthusiastically that the book helped them or their loved ones understand and endure what is often a very frightening disease. Some have told us they were spiritually transformed. For all the ways the book helped people, we are very grateful.

But we've also realized over these last four years that medicine is constantly changing, and attitudes toward life and death are also evolving. In order to make our book even more relevant, we have added sections on melanoma and ovarian cancer to chapter 4, thoroughly reworked all the medical chapters to include the latest changes in oncology, written entirely new chapters on physician-assisted suicide and hospice (chapters 14 and 15), and commented on Bill Moyers's PBS series and book *Healing and the Mind* in chapter 8.

Finally, we changed the title. *Living with Cancer* did not identify to the casual browser what was distinctive about this book—that it was the only book on the market to provide both expert medical and spiritual help for the Christian. We think *Dear God, It's Cancer* does a better job.

Thanks are due to Robert Williams, M.D., Ned Wisnefske, Ph.D., and Chriss and Douglas Ross, D.D.S., for their help on chapter 14. More thanks to Bettina Chappelle for her word-processing skills. We also owe a great debt to Janet Reed for her marvelous copyediting; she brought new life and style to our sometimes ponderous words. Our hope and prayer for this edition is that it will bring comfort and hope to those who struggle with cancer.

G.M. and B.F.
February 1997

Introduction

Why This Book?

Julie was a bit concerned when her doctor's nurse called and asked her to come in for a second Pap smear. Apparently the lab had returned positive results for her first test. What could that mean?

She found out a week later when her doctor called her in to his office to give her the results of the second test. "You have cervical cancer," he told her bluntly. "I'll schedule you for surgery as soon as possible."

Julie was so stunned she could hardly think. Her first feeling was fear—and worry. Was she going to die? She had four children, and the youngest was still nursing. How would they survive without her?

The doctor told her that since they had discovered the cancer so early, she had a good chance of recovery. But that reassurance brought on a whole new set of questions. What was "a good chance"? What kinds of treatments would she have to endure in the next months? How would she pay for them?

And where was God in all of this? Julie believed in God—but why would God allow such a thing to happen to her? There were so many questions, and so few answers.

We wrote this book to give people like Julie, along with their friends and family, honest and easy-to-understand answers to the full range of questions—both medical and spiritual—that cancer provokes.

What gives us the right to tackle these questions? Bill is a practicing oncologist (cancer specialist) who has treated cancer patients every day for years. Gerry is a professor of religion who has pastored cancer patients and their families. We have both faced cancer in our personal lives as well; both of our mothers have had cancer. We have pooled our experience and training to provide what no other book we know of provides:

- easy-to-understand explanations of the basic medical facts about cancer

- answers to the spiritual and religious questions that confront most cancer patients and their loved ones

The first part of this book is devoted to presenting, in plain language, the medical facts about cancer. Chapter 1 explains what happens when a cell becomes cancerous. Chapter 2 tells what we know about the causes of cancer. Chapter 3 provides some insights into why a doctor will schedule a battery of tests to "stage" the cancer and also explains the most important tests doctors use to determine how far a cancer has progressed. Chapter 4 provides a detailed but easy-to-understand description of the six common types of cancer in the United States: breast cancer, lung cancer, colo-rectal cancer, prostate cancer, ovarian cancer, and melanoma. And chapter 5 presents a basis for a solid understanding of the four basic types of cancer treatment: chemotherapy, surgery, radiation, and biological treatments.

Dear God, It's Cancer goes on to address some pragmatic questions that commonly arise but are seldom covered elsewhere. Irene, for instance, is ninety years old. She keeps asking her pastor why God doesn't take her home to heaven. Recently her doctor found a tumor in her breast and wants to operate. Irene doesn't want the surgery, and her family doesn't know what to do. Does Irene have the right to refuse her doctor's recommendation? Chapter 6 discusses this and other questions about the doctor-patient relationship. Chapter 7 offers suggestions on how to sort through the blizzard of paperwork involved in paying cancer-related bills.

Another pragmatic issue rarely covered in other books is that of the many alternative treatments that claim to offer help for cancer. How do we distinguish between the genuine and the counterfeit? Howard was a sixty-year-old businessman with prostate cancer. His doctor recommended hormonal therapy, but his health-food-conscious neighbor advised him to try megadoses of vitamins. One of his office associates showed him an article on coffee enemas that claimed remarkable cures. Then his wife told him about a book that promises spiritual and physical healing to those with true faith. How was he to choose a treatment? Chapter 8 attempts to sort such choices out.

If spiritual questions are most pressing for you at this time, you might want to turn first to chapter 9. Here we focus on the agonizing question most cancer patients eventually ask: Why did God allow me (or my loved one) to get cancer? If God is good and all powerful, why does he allow any suffering at all? Chapters 9, 10, and 11 suggest answers that countless cancer patients have found helpful and satisfying.

If you are searching for spiritual peace and the strength to help you cope, you'll want to turn to chapter 12. It offers a number of suggestions gleaned from patients who have been there. And if you are seeking healing for yourself or your loved one or wondering if healing is even possible, turn to chapter 13. It brings a balanced but hopeful approach to this tricky issue and tells three stories of cancer cases in which healing occurred through a combination of medicine and prayer.

When some people discover they have cancer, their first thought is to kill themselves. They remember the terrible suffering a relative endured twenty years earlier, and vow they won't go through the same experiences. Chapter 14 explains not only why physician-assisted suicide is more attractive today than it was in past years, but also why Christians should not take that option. Chapter 15 suggests the ideal alternative to physician-assisted suicide: hospice. This chapter shows why increasing numbers of cancer patients and their families have found dignity and comfort in hospice programs.

Finally, chapter 16 faces the practical and spiritual questions related to life after cancer. Pamela had ovarian cancer surgically removed and was given an optimistic prognosis (predicted outcome of treatment). The medical problem was temporarily, perhaps permanently, gone. But facing the possibility of death had given Pamela an entirely new view of life. How could she live from day to day after coming so close to losing her life? She knew she couldn't go on as before, but she didn't know where to begin to change. Chapter 16 offers some concrete suggestions that Pamela would find helpful.

If you or someone you love has cancer, this book is for you. It is designed to give you the medical information you need to face the enemy in the light rather than in the dark. It also points you to spiritual resources to help you find the strength to face whatever course the cancer eventually takes.

1

What Is Cancer?

How Good Cells Go Wrong

E ileen was devastated when she learned she had breast cancer—
and not just because of the waves of shock and fear that washed
over her and left her weak. Eileen also felt betrayed by her own body.
For sixty years she had given it the care that all the experts recommended—she had exercised fairly regularly, refrained from drinking
and smoking, and eaten a balanced diet. She had never taken the Pill
or any other hormone. What's more, no one in her family had ever
had cancer. Why had her body let her down? What had been a trusted
and responsible part of her was now threatening her life. It seemed to
be a clear-cut case of mutiny.

Eileen is like many patients who first come to my (Bill's) office.
They are flooded with a variety of emotions—fear, anger, worry, even
guilt or embarrassment—that often arise from false ideas about cancer.
That's why, regardless of the specific diagnosis, living with cancer
begins with understanding just what the disease is and how it operates.
(Eileen, for example, would be relieved to realize that many cancers

occur through no fault of the patient.) Understanding the disease begins with understanding precisely what we mean by the word *cancer*.

Cancer: A Definition

In short, cancer is the unregulated growth of previously normal body cells. As you probably remember from elementary school science, cells are the basic building blocks of the human body. Cancerous cells differ from normal cells in two ways. First, they duplicate abnormally. That is, they proliferate wildly with only one apparent purpose—to grow and spread. They often grow into and through surrounding normal tissues without regard to the needs and space requirements of those tissues.

The second way cancer cells differ from normal cells is that they become virtually immortal. Normal cells age and die. But most cancer cells, unless they run out of food, warmth, and water, will live as long as their human host lives.

Cancer, then, is the wild and virtually unending duplication of cells. How and why do these cells do this? We believe the best way to answer this question is to consider how normal cells behave.

Think about what happens when FAA investigators attempt to figure out the cause of a plane crash. Before they can discover what went wrong, these investigators must understand the normal functioning of an airplane. They cannot tell if engine noises recorded before a crash are abnormal if they don't know what normal engine noise sounds like. Similarly, we can best understand the growth of a cancerous cell by first examining the duplication and growth of a normal cell.

The Private Life of a Normal Cell

The healthy human body changes every minute of the day. Many of its billions of cells are constantly replacing themselves with carbon copies of their own making. This means that parts of the body you live in today are substantially different from the body you will inhabit, say, three days from now.

Some parts of your body are replaced faster than others. Your blood supply, skin, and hair, for instance, are completely exchanged over the course of several months. Brain and muscle tissues, on the other hand, change very little after we reach adulthood.

At the center of each body cell is the nucleus, which serves as the "brain" of that cell (see figure 1). The nucleus is like a computer bank; it contains all the information necessary for the future operations of that cell and all of its "daughter" cells—plus the information necessary for all the future operations of the billions of cells in the rest of the body. For example, the nucleus of a hair cell contains information not just for making hair, but also for making and operating every other part of the body.

Figure 1
Anatomy of a Cell

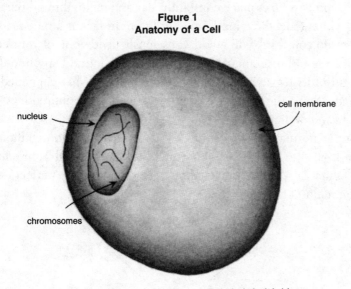

Illustration by Leah A. Johnson

This information is stored in DNA (deoxyribonucleic acid) molecules. When several thousand of these molecules are clustered to convey a piece of information, the cluster is called a gene. The particular combination of genes we inherit from our parents determines our bodies' identifying characteristics—everything from our size and shape to our hair and eye color. And the specific combination of genes is unique to each person. Even people with the same mother and father have different combinations of genetic material. Mary has blond, curly hair, for example, while her sister Jane has dark, straight hair because they each received different hair genes from Mom and Dad.

The arrangement of thousands of these genes on a strand of material is called a chromosome. Each cell in your body has forty-six chromosomes. Half of them (twenty-three) came from your mother and half (twenty-three) from your father. When the cell divides, it makes a perfect copy of all forty-six of its chromosomes (each of which has thousands of genes arranged in a precise order), then divides the surrounding tissue into exact halves and splits into two identical daughter cells.

This process takes place constantly, day and night, throughout your body without any direction from your brain. In fact, if someone asked you to, do you think you could consciously divide one of your cells? It's like the old joke about the poor centipede found lying in a ditch with all of its legs twisted together. When asked what happened, he replied, "Someone asked me how I walk with one hundred legs, and now I can't do it anymore!"

Under normal circumstances, every time one of your billions of cells duplicates, its forty-six chromosomes are perfectly reproduced (see figure 2). What happens, though, if this normally perfect duplication malfunctions?

Figure 2: Normal Cell Duplication

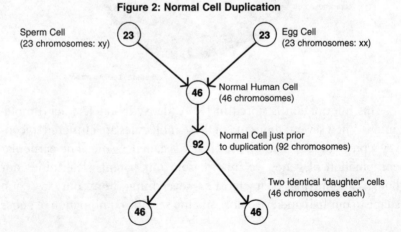

Sperm Cell
(23 chromosomes: xy) **23**

23 Egg Cell
(23 chromosomes: xx)

46 Normal Human Cell
(46 chromosomes)

92 Normal Cell just prior
to duplication (92 chromosomes)

Two identical "daughter" cells
(46 chromosomes each)

46   **46**

When Cells Go Wrong

Occasionally mistakes do occur in the normal process of cell division. Given the number of divisions that take place in a single body on any given day, a mistake or two would seem almost inevitable.

For the brief moment after the human cell has duplicated its genetic material but has not yet split into two daughter cells, ninety-two chromosomes are present at the cell. And it is in that brief moment that trouble can occur.

Suppose, for example, that one of the new daughter cells receives forty-seven chromosomes, while its sister gets only forty-five. The cell with forty-seven chromosomes might then be stronger and start crowding out its weaker sister cell. In fact, the stronger cell can develop such a growth advantage that it proliferates quickly, while its weaker sister dies and is lost forever (see figure 3).

Figure 3: Abnormal Cell Duplication

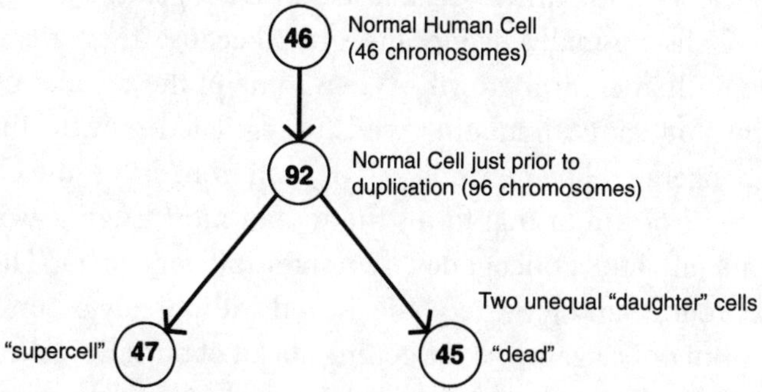

46 — Normal Human Cell (46 chromosomes)

92 — Normal Cell just prior to duplication (96 chromosomes)

Two unequal "daughter" cells

"supercell" 47   45 "dead"

Imagine what results, then, when this new "supercell" divides to become two cells, and each of those divides to produce four; the four then become eight, the eight sixteen, and so on. This explosion of abnormal cells is what produces cancer.

The How Question

But perhaps you're wondering how mistakes like these occur in the first place.

Katie wondered just that. She was in my office for a follow-up exam. Two years earlier she had noticed spots on her legs and visited her family doctor. The spots indicated lymphoma—cancer of the lymph nodes. In a short span of time Katie had gone through the shock of diagnosis, the typical battery of tests, then a course of treatment that included a bone-marrow transplant. Katie is one of the fortunate ones who survive—and even thrive—after cancer. But now she was asking the how questions—in essence, the same ones that had bothered Eileen.

How did it happen? How could my cells do this to me? Was it the nuclear power plant nearby? Was it my lab spills in freshman biology? Did I catch something from someone?

Answering these questions required me to return to the level of the gene—the small section of a chromosome that holds a particular piece of information. My explanation went something like the following.

A Closer Look at the Cellular Level: Oncogenes

Cells normally divide and grow because they are stimulated by genes that control growth. When some of these genes get out of control and start stimulating wild, unregulated growth, they are called oncogenes. (The prefix *onco* is derived from *onkos*, the Greek word for a mass or tumor that forms the root of most English words related to cancer.) These oncogenes are responsible for cancer. They tell cells to reproduce and grow too quickly and without any order.

But once again, we are getting ahead of ourselves. We need to know why oncogenes exist in the first place. What transforms a normal gene that regulates cell growth into an oncogene that breeds chaos and destruction?

What Turns a Normal Gene into an Oncogene?

This is a difficult question that scientists are only beginning to unravel. But according to our latest thinking, at least four kinds of events can lead to this transformation. These events do not completely explain what causes the cancer—or why one person develops cancer and another does not. (For a more complete discussion of that issue, see chapter 2.) But they do help us understand the transformation of a normal cell into one that is growing out of control.

Event #1: Invasion of a Virus

The first kind of event that can cause a gene to be transformed into an oncogene is the introduction of a virus into a cell. A virus is a tiny piece of DNA or RNA (ribonucleic acid, another molecule like DNA) that is capable of infecting a cell and reproducing itself. Scientists have determined that viruses are linked to at least five different types of cancer: a rare form of leukemia, cervical cancer, liver cancer, Burkitt's lymphoma (an extremely rare cancer of the lymph system), and Kaposi's sarcoma (a cancer of connective tissue associated with AIDS). Viruses have also been shown to cause cancer in animals.

Scientists now believe that the insertion of a virus into a cell may turn a gene that normally regulates cell growth into an oncogene. It may also be the process of insertion that "wakes up" a "sleeping" oncogene already inside the cell.

Now, before you put on a gas mask and hide in the basement during flu season, remember this: The vast majority of cancers in the United States are not caused by viruses, and the vast majority of viruses don't cause cancer in humans. So there's really no need to worry over whether you could catch cancer from your neighbor's virus. Although it's remotely possible, the odds against it are almost overwhelming.

Event #2: A Rearrangement of Genes

Another event that can cause oncogenes to develop is a disruption in the order of genes on a chromosome. One piece of a chromosome can break off and be fitted onto another chromosome. Or a piece of chromosome can be tipped upside down (inverted) or otherwise changed (mutated) during the complex process of cell duplication. These various changes in the order of the genes on a chromosome are referred to as *translocations*, *inversions*, *point mutations*, and *duplications*. (Again, the factors that may cause these changes will be discussed in chapter 2.)

Changes in gene order are the cause of the oncogene activation that leads to chronic myelogenous leukemia (CML), a chronic malignancy of the blood that usually occurs in older people. We now believe that this malignancy is activated when a certain gene (its name is c-abl) normally found on chromosome #9 (each chromosome has a number) is broken off and swapped with a gene normally found on chromosome #22. The resulting two chromosomes are thereafter a mosaic, or mixture, of what is normally found on them.

The important point to note here is that gene c-abl, though normally harmless, loses control. At this point the cell becomes armed and dangerous because c-abl is now an activated oncogene (or a gene with the ability to stimulate cancerous changes).

Let's use continental geography as an illustration to help make this cellular behavior more clear. Imagine an enormous earthquake that made the tip of Florida and the southern tip of South America exchange places, so that Miami would find itself intact but facing Antarctica. The misplaced Miamians would find their new environment drastically changed (colder!), and they would change their behavior accordingly (dress more warmly, to begin with). So, too, the gene c-abl finds its new location on chromosome #22 startling. The change in environment causes it to lose control and order the cell to grow madly. The unfortunate result is cancer. (Fortunately, however, this form of leukemia is treatable and sometimes curable.)

Event #3: Loss of a Suppressor Gene

Oncogene activation can also occur when a previously suppressive gene is lost. That is, there may be oncogenes that are dormant only because they are continually suppressed by another gene or gene product. Imagine a hot-air balloon that is held to the ground by tethering ropes. Once the ropes are cut, the balloon goes sailing into the sky. Similarly, some genes are kept under wraps by other genes on the chromosome. But if in the intricate process of cell replication those suppressing genes are damaged or lost, the oncogene is then released to stimulate cancerous cell growth. This occurrence is called loss of inhibition by deletion of a suppressor gene.

The best-known example of a suppressor gene is p53. Twenty-five years ago, we didn't know of its existence. But today there is tremendous excitement as scientists work furiously to try to understand it. In the last several years, journal articles on the suppressor gene have appeared at the rate of more than one thousand per year.

Why this explosion of interest? We think p53 may be one of our best defenses against the development of cancer. It has been compared to the alert office clerk who notices an error in an original document and stops the copier before it spits out 500 incorrect copies. The quick-thinking p53 gene seems to watch out for damage or errors in genetic material, and then acts to correct the problem. We're not sure how it does so, but we know that when p53 is absent, these errors proliferate. Absence or mutation of this gene is associated with many different kinds of cancer.

Event #4: Redundant Duplication of a Chromosome

Oncogenes may also be activated by the redundant duplication of a chromosome. For example, children with Down syndrome have an extra copy of chromosome #21. Although most Down children do not get cancer, they do have a slightly greater chance of getting leukemia than other children. It is believed that the presence of the extra copy of chromosome #21 may cause one of its genes to trigger cancerous growth. It may be that this gene is weak—that is, not usually likely to turn into an oncogene. But the presence of a third copy of the gene, instead of the usual two after duplication, may be what triggers its transformation into an oncogene. This is called the overamplification of a gene. Overamplification is also seen in some cancers of the breast, spinal cord, and lung.

After our long discussion of the events that could trigger the growth of cancer cells, some things began to make more sense to Katie. She knew that something had suddenly gone wrong in her cells two years earlier, when cancer had struck like a bolt out of the blue. She may never know the precise how, what, when, or where of these cell events—and she still didn't know what triggered them in the first place. But she could find comfort in knowing that cancer cells don't work by black magic and that she probably didn't catch cancer like a flu.

Why Doesn't Everyone Get Cancer?

In summary, then, cancer is the abnormal growth of cells caused by the deregulation of cells. The genes that stimulate this deregulation are oncogenes. The startling thing to realize is that we all probably have oncogenes operating on a daily basis! As our billions of cells divide over and over every day, chromosomal accidents that produce some oncogenes probably take place regularly. The real surprise, therefore, is not that some of us get cancer, but that some of us don't!

Why don't we all develop cancer? Why do only a minority of the population contract the disease? What causes some of us to get sick while others, despite the presence of oncogenes, remain relatively healthy? The next chapter will attempt to answer these questions.

2

What Causes Cancer?

Biological, Environmental, and Lifestyle Triggers

George is seventy-five years old. His doctor has just detected a spot on his lung and suspects cancer. George is not particularly surprised because he has smoked heavily since the age of eleven. When he isn't smoking, a wad of tobacco fills his cheek. What's more, two of his brothers had cancer, and he hasn't seen a doctor since his induction into the Navy in World War II. But he is surprised that the cancer took so long to show up. Why didn't he develop cancer years ago?

Medical researchers cannot answer this question precisely. They know that certain lifestyle and environmental factors (smoking and some diets, for instance) are statistically associated with cancer. But they are hesitant to identify a particular factor in a person's life as the sole cause of that person's cancer. They insist that it is risky and probably inaccurate to think that one factor causes cancer by itself.

Some recent writers, for example, blame much cancer on emotional ill health. They say that cancer is simply a cellular-level expression of emotional disturbance. And it is true, as we shall see shortly, that depression and anxiety can affect our immune system, which is one line of defense against cancer. But to say that emotional stress alone can cause cancer is terribly simplistic. If that were the case, hospital psychiatric wards would be full of cancer patients, and cancer wards would be filled with depressed people. Neither is true.

George's case illustrates the problems with the single-cause theory. If smoking were the only factor in the development of his cancer, why didn't George's cancer show up soon after he started smoking? One reason, of course, is that cancer can lie dormant for years before it makes its presence known. But another reason is that the development of cancer is often the product of several factors working together.

We can understand this by thinking in terms of raising a crop. Many different factors may be involved in producing the final harvest. One person may prepare the ground for planting. Another person may actually put the seed in the soil, and yet another may weed the crop when the first shoots appear. Sunlight and rain, insects and weeds all help determine how the crop will germinate and grow and what kind of harvest will result.

In George's case, smoking may have prepared the "soil" and even perhaps planted the "seed." But other factors, such as poor diet or exposure to asbestos or familial predisposition or emotional stress, may have been needed to let his cancer germinate and grow.

Most cancers seem to be caused not by one factor alone, but by several factors working in concert. Some factors may work earlier in a person's life to prepare some cells for malignant change, while other factors may work later to fully activate a cancerous growth. Let's look now at the most common groups of factors that researchers believe can lead to cancer.

Does Nature Make Mistakes?
Random Genetic Changes

In the last chapter we saw that when chromosomes duplicate to produce a new cell, mistakes sometimes occur. The chromosome strands can connect where they are not supposed to connect, producing a new and unusual order of genes. If the critical error occurs in the wrong place at the wrong time, a monster—the oncogene—may be unleashed.

Why do these mistakes occur? Scientists do not know. They can only say that random mistakes seem normal. From their point of view, it seems inevitable that in an organism of such enormous complexity as the human body, with billions of cells that reproduce countless times every day, there will be occasional mistakes.

From a theological point of view, we might qualify the word *random* by saying that we believe nothing can occur—even the replication of a cell—apart from God. That is, God is the ultimate power of the universe; nothing takes place without his permission. We will discuss some of these issues later.

It's Everywhere!—Environmental Factors

Other factors that can bring on cancer are agents in the environment that may or may not be under our control.

Viruses

We have already seen, for instance, that the introduction of a virus into a cell may stimulate the development of cancer. And it has been shown that infection with certain viruses may also increase a person's chances of getting certain kinds of cancer. A person with the Hepatitis B virus (HBV), for example, runs a higher-than-normal risk of developing liver cancer. Similarly, the mononucleosis virus is associated with Burkitt's lymphoma, an extremely rare cancer of the lymph nodes.

Radiation

Radiation is another environmental factor that may influence the development of cancer. We have little control over how much radiation we receive because the vast majority of our exposure comes from natural sources.

The sun, for instance, is a source of low-level radiation that, with prolonged exposure, can damage human chromosomes and thus increase the risk of skin cancer. Although it is impossible, and probably unhealthy, to avoid all exposure to the sun, it is wise to limit your exposure to sunlight, particularly if you are fair skinned, and to use a sunscreen when you are under an intense sun for more than twenty minutes. Because the incidence of melanoma has been linked to blistering sunburns, especially in childhood, it is important to protect children from overexposure.

Researchers are now discovering that radiation can enter our homes in the form of radon[1], which is a gaseous substance emitted by the soils and rocks surrounding some homes. Most soils and rocks contain uranium and radium in widely varying concentrations, and the decay of these elements leads to the release of radon into the surrounding water and air. Since radium and uranium concentrations in the rock and soil vary so widely, the danger of exposure to radon varies enormously from place to place. Homes built on rock with a high uranium content naturally have higher levels of radon.

Exposure to radon increases the risk of getting cancer because, like all sources of ionizing radiation, radon is capable of damaging human chromosomes. As we have already seen, changes in chromosomes can transform normal genes into dangerous oncogenes. Radon exposure is particularly dangerous for smokers. It is estimated that smokers who are exposed to radon are ten times more likely to contract cancer than nonsmokers exposed to the same amount of radon.

A final common source of radiation is one over which we do have a greater measure of control: X rays. Scientists have found a higher than normal rate of cancer in people given X rays decades ago for such benign conditions as enlarged tonsils and acne. The medical profession has consequently made changes in its use of X rays. Today's X rays use less radiation and are focused on more limited parts of the body. Most physicians are aware of the risks and order these tests only when they seem essential for diagnostic or curative purposes.

Environmental Pollutants

Yet another environmental factor in the development of cancer is the presence of certain pollutants or additives in air, water, or food.

Any such substance that has been shown to contribute to cancer is called a carcinogen. It is estimated that 1 to 5 percent of all cancers are related to these agents.

The improper combustion of fossil fuels (coal, oil, natural gas) and wood can produce substances such as benzopyrene, a chemical that has been shown to be a carcinogen. Tiny amounts of this carcinogen may be present in automobile exhaust, smoke from a coal-fired power plant, and even wood stoves.

Lest you consider moving your home away from a power plant or heavily traveled street, however, consider that a cigarette smoker probably inhales one thousand times as much benzopyrene as a person who lives downwind from a coal-fired power plant or on a busy street. And the chances of getting cancer from living close to a power plant are very small. There is even an increased lung-cancer risk for people who live with smokers. With so-called passive smoking, some carcinogens that the smoker exhales go into the lungs of other people in the room.

Other chemical carcinogens also find their way into our air, water, and food supplies. Some are used in manufacturing or agriculture. A few—such as chloroform and carbon tetrachloride—are found in tiny amounts in the drinking water of some cities. They are by-products of chlorine, which is used to kill bacteria in drinking water. Once again, however, because the amounts of chlorine used are very small, the chances of getting cancer from drinking water is negligible. A few chemical substances that have been linked to cancer—such as the sodium nitrate used in curing meats or saccharin used as an artificial sweetener—are actually added to our food supply.

Many chemicals in the environment, both natural and synthetic, have been linked to cancer. The list is too long to include here. And even if we had space, printing such a list could be misleading. It might imply that it is possible and practical to avoid contact with these chemicals.

In fact it is nearly impossible to avoid environmental pollutants that have been linked with cancer. Some are in our food; some are in the air we breathe and the water we drink. Some may even be in our prescription drugs. Most of these pose little actual risk of causing cancer. If we try to eliminate all of these chemicals, we will also deprive ourselves of all of their benefits—and that may prove riskier than being exposed to the chemicals in the first place.

What We Do to Ourselves: Human Behaviors

No group has asked me (Bill) to speak on how best to get cancer. If one did, I would say something like this: Use tobacco frequently in all of its forms, drink regularly and heavily, share dirty needles, and engage in promiscuous sex. And start all this early in life while working as a lifeguard on a beach.

My point is that some carcinogens are easily avoidable. Tobacco, for instance, is probably the best-known chemical cause of cancer. It is also the most deadly. Researchers estimate that 85 to 90 percent of lung cancer cases in this country are directly related to tobacco smoking. In fact, somewhere between 25 and 40 percent of all cancer deaths in the United States result from smoking. Tobacco use is related to lung, mouth, throat, esophagus, bladder, pancreas, uterine, cervical, and kidney cancers.

Simply put, the elimination of tobacco products from our world would drastically reduce the incidence of cancer. No other single change would affect so many lives in a positive way.

But tobacco use is far from the only human behavior that increases the risk of cancer. Cancers of the esophagus, throat, and liver have been linked to heavy consumption of alcoholic beverages. A high-fat, low-fiber diet can increase the risk of developing cancer in the breast, colon, endometrium, or gall bladder. And even sexual lifestyle has a relationship to cancer. Cancer of the cervix is found more commonly in those who are sexually promiscuous than in those who have a single sexual partner or are sexually inactive.

Because radiation from the sun is a factor in producing cancer, sunbathing and working outdoors for long periods without sufficient protection can greatly increase the risk of skin cancer. This is a particularly important point to observe in a time when more and more people are getting melanoma, a very dangerous form of skin cancer. Studies have proven a clear link between prolonged exposure to the sun and skin cancers, particularly in fair-skinned persons. It is no surprise that the rate of skin cancer is higher in Australia and the American Southwest.

Finally, the use of hormones is associated with an increased incidence of cancer. For example, diethylstilbestrol (DES) is a synthetic estrogen that was commonly used in the 1950s to avert the threat of spontaneous abortion. Years later it was discovered that the daughters of women who had used this hormone had a greater risk of developing cancer of the vagina.

When We Can't Fight Back: A Weak Immune System

Another factor in cancer causation may be a weak immune system. We say may because scientists do not have much hard evidence for this theory. Some observations seem to point in this direction, but our understanding of the relationship between cancer and the immune system is still somewhat speculative.

A healthy immune system may prevent many of us from getting cancer. It does so by acting selfishly. We may criticize our children for behaving selfishly, but we should praise our immune systems for acting that way. By selfish we mean that the immune system rejects anything that appears to be foreign—whether a bacterium or virus, an organ transplanted from another person, or a cell that has become malignant (cancerous). Scientists believe that the immune system may be able to tell the difference between a normal cell and a malignant cell. So when an oncogene stimulates a cell to start reproducing wildly, the body's immune system springs into action and sends a battalion of its warriors to destroy the new enemy.

Unfortunately, some immune systems are weaker than others. As we all know from experience, not everyone succumbs to infections with the same frequency or severity; some people are more susceptible to colds and flu than others. This is because each of our immune systems has a different capacity to combat the enemy—whether a virus or a cancer. Some of us, therefore, are less resistant to the threat coming from our own oncogenes. One oncogene may slip through the immune system's defenses and develop into a cancerous growth.

Why are some immune systems weaker than others? Sometimes genetics are to blame. Sometimes diseases contracted in childhood or adulthood damage the immune system. The best-known example is AIDS, as its full name—Acquired Immune Deficiency Syndrome— suggests. Predictably, we are now seeing many AIDS patients come down with an assortment of cancers. AIDS, in fact, may be a perfect illustration of how a deficient immune system may allow cancers to develop where they would not have developed otherwise.

Malnourishment or vitamin deficiency may also weaken the immune system and thus increase the risk of cancer. And some researchers believe the functioning of the immune system is affected by our emotional ups and downs. Why is it, they ask, that cold sores appear during times of stress, even though the herpes virus that produces cold sores is present in the lip nerves for most of our lives? Why does the big pimple blossom on the forehead of the young teen just before the prom? In a similar way, continued and severe emotional stress may depress the immune system to such an extent that it is unable to fight the outbreak of oncogenes as vigorously as usual.

But once again, a weakened immune system only plays a small part in the answer to the question of what causes cancer. Some people with relatively healthy immune systems still come down with cancer. Why? Here is where the other factors come into play: random genetic mistakes, unavoidable external factors, and certain human behaviors. All of these can put such pressure on a healthy immune system that it can no longer adequately protect the body from the development of cancer. A combination of several of these factors can produce so many oncogenes that even a healthy immune system becomes overwhelmed. One or more of the oncogenes slips through the body's defenses and goes on to multiply wildly. The result is cancer.

Does Cancer Run in Families?
Genetic Factors

A person's genetic heritage may also play a role in whether a person develops cancer although the extent of that role is difficult to determine. A minority of cancers are literally passed down in classic genetic patterns. Doctors simply see that some families seem to be more cancer prone than others—and certain cancers seem more likely to run in families.

Some of these genetic predispositions are fairly obvious. For instance, the risk of skin cancers for a child of Caucasian ancestry is several times that of an African-American child. Here, the genetic influence is skin pigment, which protects against the sun's rays.

A less obvious family connection is seen in breast cancer, colon cancer, and ovarian cancer, plus a host of rarer cancers; people with a family history of these cancers do seem to have a higher risk of contracting the disease. And some cancers fall into families but don't necessarily occur in the same organs. For instance, a grandmother may have had breast cancer, an uncle pancreas cancer, and a father colon cancer.

There are two basic types of inherited cancers: organ-specific cancers and different kinds of cancers concentrated in certain families. In the first, a particular kind of cancer (say, breast) occurs at higher frequency, and at younger ages, than normal throughout the family tree. For an example of this kind of inherited cancer, see chapter 4 for our discussion of BRCA-1, the oncogene in many breast cancers.

In the second form of inherited cancer, the disease occurs in many different organs and at greatly increased frequency in some families. An example of this is the Li-Fraumeni syndrome. Families with this syndrome have a genetic defect in the tumor suppressor p53, which we discussed in chapter 1. Because of this defect, Li-Fraumeni families have malignancies of many different kinds appearing all over the family tree.

Genetic or hereditary influence is a classic example of factors you cannot avoid. You can't pick your gene pool. The best advice for people who worry about their family's risk is to share that concern with their doctors and pay close attention to the guidelines in the next few pages.

The Risk Is Relative

The fact that all the factors mentioned above have been linked to cancer does not mean that they are equally dangerous. Some pose more risk than others. Simply identifying an agent that has been associated with cancer can give the impression that one-time contact with that agent will automatically produce cancer. Actually the chances of contracting cancer from that single contact may be less than one in a thousand. For this reason, a TV or newspaper story on cancer that fails to indicate the relative risk of the highlighted factor can be very misleading.

What is relative risk? It is simply a way of indicating in realistic terms just how likely a person exposed to a specific cancer-causing agent is to develop cancer. It is expressed in terms of a number computed by comparing the exposed person's risk with the risk incurred by someone not exposed to that factor.

The relative risk of a normal person without contact with any of the factors mentioned above has been designated by researchers as 1.0. A factor that doubles the risk that person will get cancer is said to have a relative risk of 2.0. When the chances of getting cancer increase three-fold, the relative risk is 3.0, and so on.

If a particular behavior—say, eating butterflies—doubles your risk of getting cancer, then the relative risk is 2.0. This means that, all other things being equal, the person who eats butterflies has twice as much chance of getting cancer as the person who does not eat butterflies—a 100 percent increase in risk. By the same token, a relative risk of 1.1 represents a 10 percent increase in risk, and a relative risk of 0.9 means a 10 percent reduction of risk.

Please remember that a 100 percent increase in relative risk does not mean that there is 100 percent chance of contracting cancer. If eating butterflies increases the risk from two per thousand (two out of every one thousand persons not eating butterflies get cancer) to four per thousand (four out of every one thousand persons eating butterflies get cancer), the risk has doubled, or increased 100 percent. But that still means that 996 of those one thousand people eating butterflies do not get cancer.

To use a more realistic example, let's say that Mary's mother had breast cancer. As we have seen, breast cancer sometimes runs in families. So when any woman has a first-degree relation—her mother, sister, or daughter—with breast cancer, that woman's relative risk is around 2.0. Mary's relative risk of also developing breast cancer, therefore, is 2.0—double that of a woman who has no family history of breast cancer. And the relative risk increases if other factors are involved. If, for example, Mary's mother or sister contracted cancer in both breasts while still a young woman (before menopause), Mary's risk of developing breast cancer would be 4.0—four times the average.

With this background, consider how a news story on breast cancer can give a false impression. Say, for example, that the story reports a link between postmenopausal estrogen use and breast cancer, but doesn't report that the relative risk of hormone use is only about 1.2. Women who have used that hormone can easily get the impression that they are doomed to develop cancer when their relative risk may actually be much lower than Mary's. If the relative risk of such hormone use is 1.2, the hormones have increased their risk by only 20 percent, as opposed to Mary's 400 percent.

The lesson to be learned from this is that some factors that contribute to cancer are more dangerous than others. Many pose minimal risk by themselves. (Table 1 shows the relative risks of the contributing factors discussed in this chapter.) And even the simultaneous presence of a number of these factors does not always lead to cancer. So you need not be unduly concerned if one or more of the factors described in this chapter pertains to you.

Can I Avoid Cancer?

As we have already seen, few of the factors discussed in this chapter have been proven to be causes of cancer. Most of them are simply linked to, or correlated with, cancer. And other factors may be involved

Table 1
Relative Risk Table
(for comparison purposes only)

Risk Factor	Cancer	Relative Risk (1.0 = No Increase)
TOBACCO	lung cancer	8.0–10.0
	esophageal cancer	7.0
	bladder cancer	2.0
ALCOHOL	esophageal cancer	1.0 if no tobacco or alcohol used 50.0 if alcohol is used heavily 150.0 if both tobacco and alcohol abused
	breast cancer	1.4–1.7
LOW DIETARY FIBER	colon cancer	exact relationship unknown
HIGH DIETARY FAT	breast cancer	1.0–2.0
	colon cancer	1.0–2.0
OBESITY	endometrial (uterine) cancer	5.0
	gall-bladder cancer	3.0
	breast cancer	1.5
	lung cancer	1.0
ESTROGEN THERAPY	endometrial cancer	8.0–16.0
	breast cancer	1.0–1.5
SEXUAL PROMISCUITY	uterine/cervical cancer	exact relationship unknown
DELAYED PREGNANCY	breast cancer	exact relationship unknown
FAMILY HISTORY OF BREAST CANCER	breast cancer	2.0 if first-degree relative has breast cancer 4.0 if first-degree relative has premenopausal cancer in both breasts
FOOD ADDITIVES	all cancers	small, unknown risk
POLLUTION	all cancers	small, unknown risk
MEDICAL X RAYS	all cancers	small, unknown risk
FLUORIDE IN WATER		no risk
SACCHARIN	bladder cancer	no proven increased risk in humans
ASBESTOS	lung cancer (mesothelioma)	3.0–4.0
SILICONE BREAST IMPLANTS		no risk*

*The problems reported in the media, allegedly associated with silicone breast implants, have nothing to do with cancer. There is no evidence that silicone implants increase the risk of cancer.

that we are not aware of. Thus avoiding certain factors will not necessarily guarantee that a person will never develop cancer. At any rate, some factors may be impossible or unwise to avoid entirely. Our genetic heritage is certainly beyond our control. X rays are sometimes necessary for medical treatment. We can minimize exposure to radiation from sunshine but not escape it without becoming reclusive, which itself is unhealthy. And some pollutants are unavoidable for most people living in industrialized societies.

But there is evidence that avoiding as many of these factors as possible will reduce the chances of developing cancer. Groups of people with different lifestyles have cancer rates that dramatically differ from the rates of people who live in the same region. Mormons in Salt Lake City, for instance, do not smoke or drink, and they have markedly lower rates of cancer than the rest of the population of Salt Lake City.

We also know that migrating peoples tend to assume the cancer rates of their new communities. Japan, for example, has a lower rate of some cancers than the United States. But when Japanese people move to the United States and adopt an American lifestyle, their chances of contracting these cancers increase.

It seems evident, therefore, that avoiding certain cancer-related factors can reduce your chances of getting cancer. And we believe it makes sense to focus on those factors you can control most easily. For example, while you cannot do a lot (in the short term, at least) to reduce the amount of chemicals in the environment, you can do a lot to change what you do with your body and mind and thereby reduce your cancer risks.

When I (Bill) first met Ben, he was as disgusted as any new cancer patient I'd ever met. Ben had religiously practiced a vegetarian diet for decades. Now he faced colon cancer surgery. He felt absolutely cheated! While his high-fiber, low-fat diet was exactly the right choice for health, he still faced colon cancer. Ben and I talked about the choices we make but that guarantees don't come with these bodies of ours. "Perhaps," I told him, "your choices prevented colon cancer's arrival until now."

What changes should you make? We suggest the following guidelines, which are healthy for anyone, at risk for cancer or not:

1. Reduce dietary fat to 30 percent of your total calories—a total daily fat intake of about 75 grams. Ask your doctor or a nutritionist for more detailed instruction on fat in different foods, and read the labels on packaged food. Most indicate the number of grams of fat contained in each serving. Be sure to pay attention to what the label considers a serving.

2. Increase fiber intake to 20 to 30 grams per day. You can get fiber from whole-grain breads and cereals and from whole-plant products such as celery, cabbage, and lettuce.

3. Eat a variety of fruits and vegetables on a regular basis. Vitamin C (found in citrus fruits), vitamin E (found in grain products), vitamin A (found in fortified milk), beta carotene (found in vegetables, particularly carrots), and selenium (also found in vegetables) may help prevent certain cancers.

4. Avoid obesity and exercise regularly. Few cancers are directly related to being obese or out of shape, but being fit enhances your ability to survive therapy and fight cancer.

5. Avoid or limit alcoholic beverages.

6. Avoid tobacco in every form.

7. Check your home for radon, especially if you are a tobacco smoker. Call your county extension agent to see if your geographical area tends to have high concentrations of this gas. If the answer is yes, a radon home test kit can be purchased at a relatively low price at some drug and hardware stores.

8. Use a potent sunscreen on yourself and your children. Avoid a blistering sunburn at all costs, especially for children.

9. Minimize your intake of salted, cured, or smoked foods. Avoid saccharin in large amounts.

10. Strengthen your emotional health (thus strengthening your immune system) by sharing your burdens with a trusted friend or family member. You may want to seek professional counseling if persistent problems are causing stress.

11. Strengthen your spiritual health by striving to be closer to God. Use prayer, worship, quiet time with God, Scripture readings, inspirational books, and the comfort of an abiding friend.

No Guarantees!

With tongue in cheek, I have told many audiences that the only certain way to reach the century mark is first to check your basement for radon. Then, if the radon level is low, you should move down there at a young age. Be sure not to go out into sunlight. Always eat organically grown vegetables and boiled white meats. Drink distilled water and totally avoid sex, alcohol, or tobacco. If you do this, I assure my audiences, you'll probably live a long time. But will it be any fun?

All this is to point out the obvious. Life is full of risks. Some are very serious; others are not. Some are unavoidable, while others are associated with lifestyles you can avoid. Equipped with this knowledge, you can now think about your own life, family history, and habits and draw up a list of New Year's resolutions to implement as soon as you are ready.

If you, or someone you love, have already been diagnosed with cancer, it may seem a little late to talk about avoiding cancer. But understanding that cancer is caused by a combination of factors should show you there's no point in second-guessing yourself. Your smoking or your diet or your sunbathing may indeed have contributed to your cancer—but so might your ancestry, life events that weakened your immune system, or other factors you could not control. Instead of beating yourself up with if onlys, your best strategy is to focus your efforts on the current situation and fight to win.

3

Has It Spread? How Far?

Tests and Procedures You Might Expect

The experience of cancer is like running a race with hurdles set up along the way to the finish line. The first, and often tallest, hurdle for the patient is discovering that he or she has cancer. That moment can be shattering—but it is far from the end of the race. The next big hurdle is facing the question: Has it spread?

The process of determining how far a cancer has advanced—what stage it has reached—is called staging. This typically takes place after a biopsy (removing and evaluating a piece of tissue to see if it is malignant) has been performed. If the tissue is malignant, the doctor will order a series of tests to determine how far the cancer has progressed. Only after these tests are done and their results are known will the doctor begin treating the cancer.

Now, the word staging can be misleading. One can get the impression that all cancers progress in similar stages—that a breast cancer in stage two would be similar to a colon cancer in stage two. This is not the case. Each type of cancer progresses in its own unique ways, and there are no stages common to all types of cancer. Nevertheless, it is often possible to estimate how far in the body a particular cancer has progressed, and this determination can be very important to the treatment and prognosis (your doctor's best guess of the expected outcome).

For example, breast cancer starts with a tiny spot and usually spreads in an orderly pattern. A breast tumor may be small and limited to one breast—that is one stage. Or it may have spread to lymph nodes under the arm—a more advanced stage. It might even have spread to other organs—a still more advanced stage. If the tumor is discovered at a very early stage, chances of recovery are excellent, and treatment will be of one sort. But if the tumor is not detected until it has spread considerably, chances of recovery are reduced, and treatment will be of a different sort. Staging enables the doctor to predict the chances of recovery and determine the best kind of treatment.

Staging is not as important for malignancies that progress in a less orderly fashion. For example, leukemia (cancer of the blood), some forms of lymphoma (cancer of the lymph system), and myeloma (cancer of the bone-marrow plasma cells) tend to spread widely because of the fluid nature of the affected tissue. Since the doctor usually cannot distinguish between the site of origin and later spread for these kinds of cancer, staging is less important for predicting the right kind of therapy. For some forms of leukemia, for example, treatment will be the same regardless of how early the cancer has been detected.

For many cancers, however—including breast, colon, ovarian, lung, and prostate cancers—staging is extremely important. The rest of this chapter, therefore, will describe the tests most commonly used in this process. They fall into four main groups:

- blood tests
- radiographic tests (pictures taken by a radiologist)
- biopsies (removing a piece of tissue for examination)
- endoscopies (ways of literally "looking inside" an organ or cavity)

We will describe each of the most common tests, what they might feel like to the patient, how they are performed, and how the doctor might use their results. First, however, we want to point out that some of these procedures are also valuable as screening devices to detect cancer at the earliest possible stage and thereby increase the possibility of cure. Table 2, American Cancer Society Cancer Screening Guidelines, lists the procedures that are valuable in this respect and suggests the situations that call for these procedures.

Blood Tests

The blood can reveal many things about a patient's condition. In order to understand just what it can reveal, let's take a minute to review some high-school biology.

Blood, you may remember, is made up of cells and their surrounding liquid. There are three types of cells: white blood cells (leukocytes), red blood cells (erythrocytes), and platelets (thrombocytes). White blood cells fight infections and help the body build up immunity to disease. Red blood cells are simply sacs of hemoglobin, a substance that carries oxygen throughout the body. Platelets are tiny particles that promote blood clotting when necessary.

The liquid part of the blood is plasma (also called serum). This is a yellow substance containing salts, minerals, and protein. Plasma studies, often referred to simply as blood studies, are very valuable for what they can tell about a patient's condition.

Blood tests obviously involve taking blood from the body—usually from the inside of the elbow or the fingertip. A needle is always involved. And yes, it hurts to get poked with a needle. How much it hurts will depend on the patient's pain threshold and on the skill of the technician taking the blood.

An aside from Bill: There are many things they didn't teach me in medical school. One is the vital importance of people called ancillary staff. These people who work in medical labs, performing tasks essential to the diagnosis and treatment of cancer, touch patients' lives many times each day. Just ask a veteran of cancer therapy about

Table 2
American Cancer Society
Cancer Screening Guidelines

Test or Procedure	Sex	Age	Frequency
Sigmoidoscopy, preferably flexible	Male & Female	50 and over	Every 3–5 years
Fecal Occult Blood Test	Male & Female	50 and over	Every year
Digital Rectal Examination	Male & Female	40 and over	Every year
Prostate Exam*	Male	50 and over	Every year
Pap Test	Female	All women who are, or who have been sexually active, or have reached age 18, should have an annual Pap test and pelvic examination. After a woman has had three or more consecutive satisfactory normal annual exams, the Pap test may be performed less frequently at the discretion of her physician.	
Pelvic Examination	Female	18–40 40 and over	Every 1–3 years with Pap test. Every year
Endometrial Tissue Sample	Female	At menopause, if high risk†	At menopause and thereafter at the discretion of the physician.
Breast Self-Examination	Female	20 and over	Every month
Clinical Breast Exam	Female	20–40 40 and over	Every 3 years Every year
Mammography‡	Female	40–49 50 and over	Every 1–2 years Every year
Health Counseling and Cancer Checkup§	Male & Female	20 and over 40 and over	Every 3 years Every year

*Annual digital rectal examination and prostate-specific antigen should be performed on men 50 years and older. If either is abnormal, further evaluation should be considered.
†History of infertility, obesity, failure to ovulate, abnormal uterine bleeding, or unopposed estrogen or tamoxifen therapy.
‡Screening mammography should begin by age 40.
§To include examination of the thyroid, testicles, ovaries, lymph nodes, oral region, and skin.
Source: American Cancer Society Screening Guidelines, published annually.

the importance of a good venipuncture tech—the person who draws a blood sample from a patient. The veteran patient will smile and tell you in no uncertain terms who is good and who is great. Oncologists— and cancer patients—owe a great debt to the ancillary staff.

Now let's take a look at why all this bloodletting is done. Blood samples are needed in order to conduct a variety of blood studies. Those most commonly used for staging are the complete blood count, chemistries, and tumor markers.

Complete Blood Count

The complete blood count (CBC), one of the most commonly used tests, measures the quantity of red blood cells, white blood cells, and platelets in a sample.

The CBC is used at the beginning as a diagnostic tool and then throughout the course of therapy to assess the patient's ability to tolerate further therapy. A veteran of chemotherapy will often follow up, "How are you, doctor?" with "What's my blood count today?" The experienced patient knows that without an adequate cell count, many cancer therapies are unsafe.

Besides telling the doctor whether the patient is able to receive chemotherapy, the CBC also predicts the risk of unwanted bleeding or serious infection and indicates the need for blood transfusions.

Chemistries

Chemistries sound like something out of high-school laboratory days, but it is actually a measurement of important salts, minerals, and proteins contained in the blood plasma (serum). From these measurements, doctors learn about kidney and liver function; about the levels of body salts, cholesterol, and blood sugar; and about the balance between acids and bases in the body. Test results will indicate the quantities of such substances as potassium, creatinine, liver enzymes, and albumin. These results help the physician know how well the parts of the body are performing their daily tasks. They also help to predict how well the patient will tolerate further therapy.

Tumor Markers

A cancer cell may produce a variety of proteins and other substances that can be directly measured in the bloodstream. Doctors call these tumor markers because they mark the presence or absence of a tumor. They enable the physician to monitor tumor activity both at the beginning of diagnosis and throughout the course of therapy, then to assess the patient's response to treatment. Here are descriptions of the most important tumor markers in the blood.

- Lactate dehydrogenase (LDH) is an enzyme (body protein), the amount of which greatly multiplies in such diseases as lymphoma, Hodgkin's disease (a form of lymphoma), and germ cell tumors (cancer of either the testicles or ovaries). Changes in LDH levels are watched very closely in these cancers because they often mirror their growth and remission.

- Alpha fetoprotein (AFP) is a protein normally produced by fetal tissue (while the baby is still in the womb). In the healthy body, it is no longer needed after birth, and blood levels fall during the baby's first year. But certain tumors, such as in liver cancer and germ cell cancers, begin to produce this protein again. Measuring AFP in the blood helps doctors to diagnose these cancers as well as to observe response to treatment.

- Human chorionic gonadotropin (Beta HCG) is a hormone normally produced in large quantities only by the placentas of pregnant women. But cancers, particularly those of the ovary or testicle, can also produce high levels of this hormone. Its rise and fall in the bloodstream can be monitored to keep track of tumor activity.

- Carcinoembryonic antigen (CEA) is another protein that is normally found in small amounts in the bloodstream. It has no proven function in adult life but was probably valuable when we were embryos in the womb—hence the name. However, its level may rise markedly in the presence of cancer of the liver, lung, breast, or colon. It, too, is valuable both for diagnosis and monitoring.

- Abnormal immunoglobulins manufactured by malignant lymph cells known as plasma cells are measured by a process called immunoelectrophoresis (IEP). IEP is most helpful in multiple myeloma (when these plasma cells have become malignant in several bones). A rise or fall in abnormal immunoglobulins corresponds to the growth or remission of multiple myeloma.

- Prostate-specific antigen (PSA) is made only in prostate tissue and can be elevated by both benign (noncancerous) and malignant conditions. A very high level of PSA is often indicative of cancer within the prostate gland. This test is used along with digital examination, ultrasound, and biopsy to diagnose prostate cancer. (Prostatic acid phosphatase—or PAP—is another tumor marker in patients with prostate cancer.)

- Alkaline phosphatase is an enzyme manufactured by normal bone cells, white blood cells, and bile ducts. Changes in levels of alkaline phosphatase in the plasma may be signs of a malignant tumor invading the liver or bone. Doctors test for levels of this enzyme not to determine treatment, but to get an idea where to look for further spread of cancer.

- Miscellaneous proteins are manufactured by the body in the presence of cancer that are found only in low levels in people without cancer. These proteins have no known purpose in the healthy body and have been given numbers for the purpose of further study. The three most important of these are CA15-3, CA19-9, and CA-125. CA15-3 (also called 27.29 by some laboratories) is found in some breast-cancer patients, while CA19-9 is found in patients with various intestinal cancers, especially in cancers of the pancreas. CA-125 is an ovarian cancer protein that can be elevated in the presence of both benign and malignant abnormalities of the female organs, but is especially high in the case of ovarian cancer.

All of these blood tests—blood counts, chemistries, and tumor markers—provide invaluable assistance to the physician who is trying to put together the jigsaw puzzle of a patient's cancer treatment. But the blood tests are only the first step. A patient needs other tests as well—such as radiographic studies.

Radiographic Studies

The radiology suite will likely become a familiar place to patients diagnosed with cancer, and its staff will become close acquaintances. The radiologist and his or her various machines are essential to diagnosis and staging, as well as in some forms of treatment. The following are the most important tests conducted by radiologists and their staff.

X-Ray Studies

This form of radiographic study was among the first ever developed in the medical field, so it is the best understood by most patients. X rays are tiny beams of energy capable of passing through human tissue. They are useful to us because tissues and organs have different densities and so allow penetration of X rays to different depths. When X rays are aimed through human tissue and used to expose special film, tissues of different densities will have different shading on the completed picture. Because tumors are usually of greater density than their surrounding tissues, they stand out clearly in the X-ray picture.

A good example of this is the spot on the lung. For years, doctors have been able to detect lung cancer by observing a relatively dense lung tumor standing out against the low-density lung tissue that surrounds it. On the X ray, the tumor appears white against a dark background of lung tissue.

Typically, a simple X ray is painless. Some of the more complex procedures (described below) may involve some discomfort.

CAT Scan

The CAT (Computerized Axial Tomography) scan is another, much more sophisticated form of X ray. It is a computer-generated picture that gathers the X-ray information, processes it, and then reassembles the information in three-dimensional form. CAT scans give doctors remarkable views of the inside of the human body—as if the body had been sliced and the pieces laid out flat on a table for them to view. Tumors as small as a green pea can often be detected. The CAT scan has significantly advanced physicians' ability to stage cancers as well as helping them better understand a host of other illnesses.

The CAT scan can be very useful in follow-up exams. Let me give you an example. Willard is a seventy-five-year-old gentleman who was never sick a day in his life—until he noticed a bit of blood on the toilet paper. Shortly afterward, his colon cancer was removed, along with some lymph nodes in the area, which were also found to contain cancer cells. But while his surgeon removed all the cancer he could see, he wasn't sure that Willard was completely clear.

A year later something was wrong. Willard had received twelve months of chemotherapy, but the level of his CEA protein was rising. This told me (Bill) that a small cluster of cancer cells had survived somewhere in Willard's body. But where? No tests were able to detect the location of these cancer cells until I ordered a CAT scan for Willard. Then we found a malignant cluster in his liver and removed them by surgery. Six years later Willard still poses a severe threat to the wild turkey population of central Virginia!

The modern CAT scan involves lying still on a flat table that slides on a dolly into a machine that resembles a large cylinder. Patients may be given an intravenous injection of dye (an image enhancing contrast material) to make the scan easier to read. This procedure may involve some discomfort in the form of a needle, an odd feeling from the dye, and even claustrophobia while in the machine. Generally, however, the process is not considered painful.

Magnetic Resonance Imaging

Magnetic Resonance Imaging (MRI) is another relatively new procedure that radiologists frequently use to help them see a cancer's growth. Instead of using X rays to see inside the body, MRI uses a giant magnet to make beautiful pictures of the inside of the body by reorienting the body's atoms.

Every part of the body is made up of atoms with electrons in orbit.

By changing the body's magnetic field with a huge and powerful magnet, and then adding pulses of radio waves, the MRI device changes the ways in which those electrons travel. Even tiny changes in the movement of these electrons are detected by the MRI scanner, and these changes are then interpreted by the computer to create intricate, breathtaking pictures of an inner organ or cavity.

The advantages of MRI are twofold. Since it is not an X ray, the very small risk of radiation is eliminated entirely. As far as we know, the magnetic fields used by MRI do not damage the body in any way. MRI is also beneficial because of the detailed pictures it gives, especially of the bone marrow and the central nervous system.

Like the CAT scan, an MRI can involve some discomfort to the patient. There is often an injection of a contrasting agent, and the same problem of claustrophobia may exist. I have also been told that the MRI machine is very noisy and that some patients find this unpleasant. A new generation of open MRIs has been developed that are less likely to cause claustrophobia.

In some cases, these beautiful pictures can tell too much; they are difficult to interpret. I can't help but think of Maria, who underwent a bone-marrow transplant for multiple myeloma. For her follow-up testing, I ordered an MRI of her bone marrow. The MRI dutifully pictured everything it saw inside her bones, which included a large number of holes. The report I received read, "Multiple deposits of recurring myeloma."

It was hard for me to give Maria the bad news. I wasn't sure what the picture meant, but I told her that we needed to do a bone-marrow biopsy to be sure. To my delight, the bone-marrow biopsy (a microscopic analysis of actual bone marrow) showed only healthy marrow! In this case, the MRI had done its job. The innumerable holes it showed were there. But these weren't cancerous holes; they were cavities filled with recovering, transplanted marrow.

The MRI gives us marvelous pictures, indeed, but what these pictures mean is not always clear. In this case Maria had to endure what turned out (in hindsight) to be an unnecessary test. She agrees with me, however, that it was better to be safe than sorry.

Ultrasound

Another test that avoids all risk of radiation is the ultrasound, which uses sound waves to take its pictures. These photographs enable radiologists and oncologists to distinguish among solid, hollow, and fluid-filled structures. Ultrasound is particularly valuable because it can look through liquid tumors and the fluid-filled parts of the body such as the urinary bladder. Radiologists often use it to determine whether a mass is a benign cyst (filled with fluid) or a malignant tumor (usually solid). Oncologists are especially likely to order ultrasound when looking at the pelvis, the kidneys, the liver, and the female breast.

Pain is not common with wave tests like the ultrasound. Patients may be asked to keep their bladders almost unbearably full, however, because this makes the visual image clearer for the doctor.

Barium Evaluations

A barium evaluation is an X-ray procedure that involves filling a part of the stomach or intestine with a contrast liquid (patients often think of this as a dye) that X-ray beams cannot penetrate. By putting this liquid into the stomach, for instance, and shooting an X ray at the region, the radiologist can see a direct outline of the stomach. These pictures can be taken either as snapshots or motion pictures. The latter are helpful in assessing the process of swallowing and digestion and monitoring ulcers and some tumors. A barium enema is used to accurately outline the colon and rectum in ways not possible with a simple X ray.

The X-ray procedure in these barium tests is not painful, but getting barium inside can be. First, the intestine is cleared with vigorous laxatives, then the barium is squirted into the rectum. This can be uncomfortable, not to mention a bit embarrassing.

Nuclear Medicine

Nuclear testing also uses radiation, but not from a machine outside the body. Instead, radioactive chemicals are injected into a patient's vein and then scanned as they circulate through the body. The radiologist has a choice of several chemicals whose molecules are attracted to certain kinds of tissue. A radiologist looking for bone cancer, for instance, will use a chemical that has a propensity to seek out bone. In what is called a bone scan, the radiologist will be able to detect signs of tumors in bone tissue—in an arm, leg, rib, or spine—by seeing where these chemicals land. Radiologists looking for other kinds of cancer will use other radioactive chemicals that are drawn to the organ they wish to investigate. This nuclear fox hunt is most effective for looking at cancers of the liver, lymph nodes, brain, and spleen.

In the next few years, we are likely to see the emergence of a new generation of nuclear tests for cancer and other diseases. Other tests can tell us how the shape or size or density of a tumor has changed, but none of them (not even a CAT scan) can look into the working mechanisms of a tumor to determine if it is alive or dead. Now, however, PET (Positron Emission Tomography) scans are able to do just that. They are already in use as research tools, and are used to test patients at some large hospitals.

PET scans will help an oncologist determine if a tumor is growing or dead by looking at its glucose (sugar) intake. If the tumor is using glucose (taking in more of it than surrounding tissue), we can assume it is alive and growing. If it is not consuming glucose, it is probably dead. We are only beginning to discover how PET scanning can help us, but the possibilities for the future are exciting.

Don't let the word *nuclear* scare you here. The actual amount of radiation used in the nuclear medicine department is usually much smaller than that in a typical X-ray test. And aside from the injection of the radioactive tracer, nuclear tests don't hurt.

Mammography

A mammogram is simply an X ray of the breast that can indicate the presence of a tumor. It is often used for screening—to detect possible tumors in breasts that show no overt symptoms of cancer—as well as to examine breasts that show symptoms such as lumps, nipple discharge, or unusual tenderness. It can be very useful in guiding biopsies of suspicious areas and helping physicians locate tumors too small to be felt by the fingers.

As development of this test has progressed, smaller and smaller tumors can be detected, treated, and removed. This procedure has greatly increased a woman's chances for early diagnosis and subsequent recovery. Although mammograms are highly accurate, they are not foolproof; some tumors do not show up. Mammography should always be used in conjunction with the patient's self-examination and the physician's exam.

Even a properly done routine mammogram may hurt. The breast is best seen when flattened some by the X-ray equipment. I've been told it can be uncomfortable.

Mammography will probably change in the near future as a new generation of ultrasound, MRI, and PET scanning becomes widely available. Some of these newer tests are already being used for high-risk women whose breasts are difficult to image with conventional mammography. Ask your doctor if you think this may apply to you.

Biopsies—"What, More Needles?"

Biopsy is the only way to know for certain if someone has cancer. This is so important that it bears repeating. The only way a doctor can be absolutely sure that you have cancer is to do a biopsy—to remove a small piece of tissue from a tumor or a suspicious area and examine that tissue under a microscope.

How is the tissue obtained? Often this can be done with a surgical knife or a needle aspirate (a needle that sucks the tissue into it). Other biopsies are obtained by snaring tissue with a wire loop or fine brush.

Today's methods offer a vast improvement over biopsies done just a decade or two ago. Armed with powerful radiographic tools such as ultrasound and CAT scans, physicians can now use a needle to obtain tissues that not too long ago required major surgery to reach. Of course, some tumors are still too deep to reach or too hard to penetrate with a needle aspirate. In those cases, surgery is the only way to obtain a biopsy.

Even after the diagnosis has been made by biopsy, further biopsies may be done as part of staging. Descriptions of six common kinds of biopsies follow.

Pleural Fluid Biopsy

Pleural fluid is a liquid, present in small amounts, that bathes the outside of the lungs to keep them moist and smooth as they move within the rib cage. An increase in this fluid can indicate any of a number of cancers (lung, breast, colon, and ovarian), as well as several noncancerous conditions (tuberculosis, pneumonia, heart failure). A needle biopsy of this fluid can help diagnose the condition and also predict whether the cancer (if it is cancer) can be cured by surgery.

A pleural fluid biopsy is done with a needle—sometimes small, sometimes larger, depending on the size of specimen needed. A local anesthetic lessens, but doesn't eliminate, the pain.

Peritoneal Fluid Biopsy

Peritoneal fluid is the substance that normally surrounds the abdominal organs. An increase in its quantity can indicate the presence of ovarian or intestinal cancer. If cancer in that region is suspected, physicians will usually request a needle biopsy.

Examination of the peritoneal fluid also helps determine whether surgery would be helpful. For example, if cancer is in only one small area of the colon and has not entered the peritoneal fluid, surgery could cure the cancer. If the cancer has entered the peritoneal fluid, however, surgery will be of limited usefulness and other forms of treatment will be preferable.

This biopsy is also done with a needle and a local anesthetic. It usually hurts only a little.

Spinal Fluid Biopsy

A long chamber surrounding the spine is filled with fluid that bathes the spinal cord and brain. Tumors of the central nervous system and certain leukemias may often be detected and staged with a procedure called a spinal tap, in which spinal fluid is removed with a needle for analysis.

The procedure involves the use of a long, narrow needle, which is introduced into the space between the vertebrae, again with local anesthetic. When the chamber of spinal fluid is entered quickly and easily, pain is minimal. But when the spine is degenerated or nerves are inadvertently touched, pain can be intense.

Bone Marrow Biopsy

Analysis of the bone marrow is crucial in leukemias, lymphomas, multiple myeloma, and certain conditions such as anemia or low blood counts. The bone marrow, where all blood is manufactured, is the soft center of a bone, safely encased in its hard white exterior. To obtain a bone-marrow aspirate, the physician passes a needle through the hardened white bone to reach the soft marrow. The marrow specimen is then examined under the microscope to see if it is malignant.

Bone marrow is usually sampled just above the buttocks, in the large pelvis bones. Local anesthetic can make the skin and the bone surface numb, but the procedure still hurts. Passing a rather large needle through bone can't help but be unpleasant, and some patients request (and deserve) a sedative for this one.

Lymph Nodes

Because many cancers spread via the lymph system, a sampling of lymph node tissue can be very important to diagnosing and staging cancer. Removing an entire lymph node is a surgical procedure, usually done in an operating room. Tissue can also be removed from a lymph node by needle. It is then examined under a microscope for the presence of cancer cells.

Sometimes a lymph node is the original site of the cancer; in this case, the cancer is called a lymphoma. More often, the lymph node is merely a stopping place for circulating cancer cells as they spread from one place to another. Removing the lymph nodes, therefore, can be a treatment in itself (because it removes malignant tissue) as well as a tool for diagnosing and staging cancers.

The lymph system is one of three major networks of vessels in the body. The first is the system of arteries, which carry blood away from the heart. The second is the network of veins, which carry blood back to the heart after it has served its purpose. The third network is the lymph system, whose vessels carry a yellowish fluid that circulates at a snail's pace through our arms, legs, abdomen, chest, and head. A lymph node is a small, oval structure through which lymph fluid is filtered. There are hundreds of lymph nodes scattered throughout the body.

The lymph system carries white blood cells and drains waste products, but it can also be an avenue for the spread of cancer cells. The cancer can invade a lymph vessel near its site of origin and from there travel through the lymph system to other parts of the body.

Papanicolaou Test (Pap Smear)

A Pap smear is a very common screening biopsy used to look for signs of cancer on the uterine cervix (mouth of the womb). It is usually done during routine pelvic exams to detect any inflammation or early malignant cells of the uterus.

A Pap smear is collected by the doctor or a nurse during a pelvic examination by scraping the surface of the cervix. While the procedure can be somewhat uncomfortable, the usual complaint I hear is not pain, just the indignity of having it done.

Endoscopy—The Inside Story

The word *endoscopy* means "to look inside." Today's physicians are able to take a far deeper and clearer look, often without surgery, than they could just a few years ago. Fiber optics has made the difference— and that difference is revolutionary.

Just a few years ago, endoscopies were limited to those procedures that could be done with a rigid tube and the naked eye. This endoscope was unable to penetrate very deeply into body cavities. The modern endoscope, however, is based on fiber optics and is far more versatile. After it is inserted into the body, light passes through its optical fibers and allows the doctor to see an image, either magnified by a lens or on a video camera. Running parallel in the scope are canals through which a doctor can suction, inject, cauterize, snare tissue with a wire loop, or biopsy using a needle. Using these devices, it is possible to see clearly into dimly lit places, literally look around corners, take biopsies of tissues deep inside of the body while observing the procedure, and even cure some small tumors without surgery.

Let me give you an example of the power of these new tools. When the right lung of one of my young patients collapsed, we inserted a tube to reexpand his lung, but the lung kept deflating whenever we tried to remove the tube. Carter is a brave young man, one of Roanoke College's finest, but enough was enough.

Apparently there was a hole somewhere in the lung that would not heal. We had to find it. But how?

A surgeon on our team decided that if he could find the hole with his fiber-optic scope, he could probably repair it with a mini-incision. The surgeon found the hole and repaired it, and Carter went home the next day—thanks to fiber optics.

Let's look at eight endoscopic procedures that specialists use with cancer patients. In each of them, the basic procedure is similar although the way the scope is introduced into the body may vary. When the scope is passed through an existing body opening—for instance a nose, mouth, or anus—the pain is minimal and sedation is almost always used. Many people don't remember the experience. In the few instances when the scope must be passed through an incision, general anesthesia is used. Afterward the incision may be sore, like any other healing wound.

Bronchoscopy

A bronchoscope is used to look inside the lungs. While the patient is under sedation, a surgeon or pulmonologist (lung specialist) passes the device down the windpipe and into either lung, both to look at and to biopsy parts of the bronchial tree. Both benign and malignant conditions can be diagnosed easily with the flexible bronchoscope.

Esophagogastroduodenoscopy (EGD)

This terribly long word actually names the parts of the body at which the endoscope can look during this procedure: the esophagus (swallowing tube), the gastric region (stomach), and the duodenum (first part of the small intestine). The scope is passed through the mouth, down the esophagus, and into the region of the stomach and small intestines. EGD is used both to detect and to biopsy tumors in these regions. It is also used to look at noncancerous conditions such as peptic ulcer disease.

Endoscopicretrogradecholangiopancreatography (ERCP)

Can you believe the length of this word? It refers to a procedure in which the physician uses the EGD device described above but also introduces a dye, such as barium, into the biliary tree. The biliary tree is the series of canals that drain bile from the liver into the intestine. Tumors can either begin in the biliary tree itself or start in the pancreas and then spread to the biliary tree. By combining X-ray studies with the EGD procedure, a physician can get an accurate view of the liver, bile ducts, pancreas, and duodenum.

Using EGD and ERCP, the doctor can also find obstructions and insert small catheters (tiny tubes) to help drain around them. This procedure is used to treat obstructive jaundice, which is a common problem patients face when tumors invade the pancreas, for example. The tumor causes bile to build up in the bloodstream, which in turn gives a yellowish tint to the skin. A doctor can sometimes solve this problem by using an endoscope to insert a stent (a bypass catheter) to reroute the bile around the obstruction. This relieves the jaundice.

Colonoscopy

Colonoscopy is easy to guess from its name. It simply means looking into the colon with an endoscope that has been passed into the anus. A smaller version of this procedure is called a sigmoidoscopy, which uses a shorter instrument (it extends about two feet) and so can be performed in a doctor's office. Colonoscopy equipment is much longer and requires more expertise and greater sedation, along with more preparation of the bowel prior to the study. It is usually performed at a hospital or clinic with special equipment. The colonoscopy is performed to investigate abdominal pain, look for sites of intestinal bleeding, detect polyps and cancer, and sometimes to remove them.

Cystoscopy

Cystoscopy is usually performed by a urologist, a surgeon who specializes in the bladder and kidney. A cystoscope is passed through the urethra into the bladder (the muscular sac that collects urine) in order to look at the bladder walls from the inside. This procedure is usually done in the doctor's office and is used to investigate bladder tumors as well as benign diseases.

Colposcopy

The colposcopy scope is another invaluable application of fiber optics. A lighted tube is passed through a woman's vagina to view the female organs. The procedure is always performed by a gynecologist. The scope magnifies the tissues so the gynecologist can examine and diagnose changes in the uterus and vaginal walls. Both benign and malignant conditions can be diagnosed and treated using this technique.

Mediastinoscopy

The mediastinum is the space in the chest cavity between the lungs. There are many important structures in this part of the body — the great blood vessels, the esophagus, lymph glands, and the windpipe. The wonderful thing about mediastinoscopy is that it has largely eliminated the need to perform chest surgery just to get a look at these organs and to biopsy suspected tumors. Instead, the surgeon in the operating room passes the scope beneath the breastbone through a very small incision between the collarbones (anesthesia is always used). From there, the scope can be maneuvered to take a sample of lymph nodes for a biopsy in preparation for surgical treatment of cancer of the lung or esophagus.

Laparoscopy

Laparoscopy means "to look inside the abdominal (peritoneal) cavity." The procedure is usually done using "belly button" surgery. A small incision is made below the navel, and the lighted tube is inserted through it into the peritoneum, the cavity surrounding the abdominal organs. Through this scope, a very large area can be viewed, and both fluid samples and biopsies can be taken for diagnostic purposes. Surgeons and gynecologists use this method to detect benign conditions such as endometriosis and adhesions (scars) as well as malignant tumors. They also use this procedure to perform tubal ligations (when a woman has her Fallopian tubes "tied.")

In this chapter we have looked at the tests a physician may use to stage a patient. To determine if a cancer has spread—and how far—the physician will use blood tests, radiographic studies, biopsies, and/or endoscopies. These tests may also be used over the course of treatment to trace the progression of the disease. All along, the hope of everyone concerned is that eventually the tests will reveal good news—no more trace of cancer!

4

What Kind
of Cancer Is It?

Six Common Types of Cancer

Cancer comes in a myriad of forms, and some of these forms are so different that using the same word for all of them can be misleading. Some types of cancer, for instance, are nearly always fatal, but others are almost universally curable. When you hear the word *cancer*, therefore, you should hold off on making assumptions until you get more facts; anything you assume could be true for one kind of cancer but totally false for another.

In this chapter, we discuss six common forms of cancer: breast, lung, prostate, intestinal (colon and rectal), ovarian, and skin. Each one strikes thousands of people each year in the United States. These six kinds of cancer account for more than half of all cancers diagnosed each year on the North American continent. Beyond these, of course, there are hundreds of other forms of cancer, each with its own characteristics and treatment. Although it is impossible for a book of this size to discuss each in detail, the discussion that follows should help the majority of people dealing with cancer.

If the cancer that has disrupted your life is not one discussed here, you won't hurt our feelings if you decide to fast-forward to chapter 5. However, reading this chapter might still give you insight into how doctors often proceed when confronting cancer and what kinds of decisions you may face in deciding on treatment. Your doctor, of course, will be your best source of information regarding your particular form of cancer. In addition, the appendix lists some organizations that may be able to provide you with more information.

Breast Cancer

In the next year 180,000 women (and a few men) in the United States will discover that they have breast cancer. For some, the first sign may be a lump or feeling of tenderness in the breast area. Others, who have no symptoms, may hear the news only after a mammogram. Though the diagnosis will be a shock, there is good news for these people. Because of advanced medical treatments, the majority of individuals diagnosed with breast cancer will be alive and well five years later.

Most breast cancer is of the ductal variety. This is a fancy term for a cancer that begins in one of many breast ducts (tubes). Think of the breast duct as a long, hollow tube that connects milk-producing lobules (small clusters of glands) with the nipple. Breast cancer can also begin anywhere else in this system, from the lobule to the nipple. For example, lobular carcinoma originates in the lobules. Breast cancer of the nipple is also called Paget's disease.

If a cancer forms inside the duct or lobule and is so small that it cannot be seen from the outside, it is then an *in situ* (literally, "on the site") carcinoma (cancer). If the cancer has broken through the walls of the tube and has become visible from the outside, it is known as an infiltrating or invasive cancer. Of the two kinds (*in situ* and invasive), invasive is more dangerous.

In situ cancers of the breast, both ductal and lobular, have a very high cure rate and are treated surgically. In fact, they often require no further treatment. Nearly 100 percent of *in situ* cancers of the breast will be in remission five years later.

Invasive cancers, on the other hand, which can be very small (found only by mammography screening) or very large (a palpable lump or even as large as the breast itself), require more extensive treatment. Their rates of remission vary widely. These are the breast cancers that we will discuss in the pages that follow.

Causes of Breast Cancer

We know of a number of factors that increase the risk of getting breast cancer. Since there is so much to say about genetics, we'll briefly list the nongenetic factors first, and then discuss genetics.

- Age. The older you get, the higher the risk, starting at about age twenty.

- Geography. Women in the Western world are at higher risk than women in Asia or Africa.

- Prior history. Women who have had breast disease or a biopsy that has shown excessive growth in a duct (usually called hyperplasia or proliferative changes) are at greater risk. These growths are not malignant but sometimes develop into malignant tumors.

- Menstrual history. Generally speaking, any behavior in women that increases the uninterrupted cycle of menstruation will increase risk. Women who have never been pregnant, or become pregnant only late in life, or have had very few pregnancies, or have not breast-fed infants have higher risk. The fewer menstrual cycles in a woman's life, the better.

- Oral hormone replacement therapy (Estrogens). Now this one is tricky. There are about as many articles showing increased risk as articles showing no risk to breast tissue. The jury is still out on this one.

- Dietary fat. The more of it, the greater the risk. Fat increases the chances of breast cancer as well as the risk of heart disease and stroke. Fat is out; fiber is in.

Genetics

It should come as no surprise to anyone from a cancer-prone family that cancer can be hereditary. While it is still more common for a patient to tell me that cancer does not run in the family, the incidences of hereditary cancers are striking. For example, a forty-five-year-old woman came to see me because of a newly diagnosed cancer in her right breast. While that news was frightening enough, even more alarming was the report that her oldest sister had died recently while in her fifties with bilateral (both sides) breast cancer, and her other sister was in the last stages of her fight against bilateral breast cancer. Of the six breasts in three sisters, five were malignant, so we elected to remove the sixth as a preventive measure. This brave women has done well, but it hasn't been easy, and now she carries with her a fear of what might happen to her two daughters.

Geneticists began to look at such families many years ago, but only in the last decade have they been able to understand precisely what is passed down through the generations. The key, they have discovered, is a problem in what is called the germ line, which refers to the genetic information handed down to us from Mom's and Dad's seed, or germ. The defects in the genetic information are contained in each and every cell of the affected individual's body. These defective genes are passed on in the sperm or egg of the parent to the cells of their children.

Only about 10 percent of all breast cancers are familial, that is inherited from the germ line. The other 90 percent are the result of sporadic mutations in a single cell, which then multiplies explosively to create a tumor. In these 90 percent, the defect is limited to the tumor cells and is not passed down to children. But in the 10 percent that come from the germ line, the genetic defect is carried by every cell in the body. So when a child is born to this parent, there is a 50 percent chance (since only half of its genes come from each parent) that the child will inherit the same genetic defect in all of its cells. Researchers have now discovered several defective germ-line genes that produce breast cancer. The best known are BRCA-1 and BRCA-2

(BRCA stands for breast cancer). BRCA-1 is carried on chromosome #17, and is linked to both breast and ovarian cancer—perhaps as many as 5 percent of all cases. In fact, families with the BRCA-1 gene not only have more breast cancers than average, but more ovarian, colon, and prostate cancers as well. So this defective gene wreaks different kinds of cancer havoc. When a woman has BRCA-1 in her family tree, she worries, knowing that up to 90 percent of affected individuals may eventually develop breast cancer, and up to 50 percent get ovarian cancer in their lifetime. BRCA-2 is on chromosome #13, and causes breast cancer in both men and women. It is also linked to ovarian cancer. Researchers are working hard to figure out exactly how these genes cause cancer. If they discover the mechanism, the payoffs for predicting and treating cancer should be enormous.

Genetic Testing: The Bad News

Now that cloning (reproducing a segment of DNA, the genetic material) is possible, it is also possible to test for the presence of defective genes in high-risk families. This may sound like great news. But there are dangers involved, which Dr. Mark Greene of the Mayo Clinic Scottsdale recently described in the Mayo Clinic Proceedings.[1] I have paraphrased his discussion as follows.

Before consenting to any kind of testing for a genetic defect, a patient should have the chance to think through and perhaps discuss with a physician the following points:

- A blood test—and for that matter any kind of test—can give false positive or false negative results. Breast cancer gene testing is no different. When falsely negative, it can lead to unwarranted joy; when falsely positive, to unnecessary worry.

- Responsible doctors consider genetic counseling a must. This kind of counseling, which advises patients on what to do if they discover they have higher genetic risks, costs money and is not always covered by insurance.

- The burden of testing positive may be difficult to bear, both psychologically and spiritually.

- It may be difficult to get health and life insurance (not to mention a job) if a positive test becomes known. It may be difficult even if it is only another member of the family who carries the genetic defect. As of this writing, genetic privacy is not guaranteed by the laws of the land.

- We can now test for two genes that produce breast cancer, but there may be many more that we have not yet discovered.

- Doctors and hospitals always intend to keep medical records private, but with more and more records going into computers, more and more people have access to that information.

- It is easy to imagine situations in which some members of a family will want the entire family to get genetic testing, and others won't. This could ignite a difficult and possibly divisive quarrel.

- Testing is expensive, even more so when several members of a family are tested.

- Perhaps most important, there is still no conclusive evidence that testing helps anyone in the long run. There are no long-term studies to help us know what to recommend to high-risk families when they are discovered. It is possible, of course, that this information could lead to preventive mastectomies, hormone treatments, and very careful use of mammography.

Genetic Testing: The Good News

Those are the dangers of genetic testing. You can see that testing should not be taken lightly. But there may be advantages to finding out if you have the BRCA-1 or BRCA-2 genes. You can then have accurate information about your increased risk, which means you can think about whether preventive removal of breast tissue might benefit you. You will probably be more vigilant about examining your breasts and getting mammograms. And you may pay closer attention to your diet, eating less fat and more fiber, and your exercise regimen.

On the other hand, getting tested and finding out that you are negative (free of a defective gene) will probably relieve you of several fears—that you might have to consider preventive removal of your breast or ovaries, or that your abnormal gene will be passed on to your children.

I have presented this information about genetic testing both to inform you of the latest developments and to help you think twice before you rush to request genetic testing. It is appropriate for the following persons to consider genetic testing.

- Women who had breast cancer diagnosed before age thirty.

- Women who had breast or ovarian cancer diagnosed before age fifty and have a first-degree relative (sister, mother, or daughter) who had breast or ovarian cancer diagnosed before age fifty.

- Women who had breast cancer and whose family has had two or more cases of breast cancer and one or more cases of ovarian cancer.

- Women who have a first-degree relative (mother, sister, or daughter) who is known to carry the BRCA-1 or BRCA-2 gene.

- Ashkenazi Jewish women with breast cancer diagnosed before age forty, or ovarian cancer diagnosed at any age. This ethnic group carries a higher risk of these mutations.

One last word about genetic testing. The American Society of Clinical Oncology has urged its doctors who order these tests to encourage their patients to participate in long-term outcome studies, so we can learn more about genetic cancers.

Treating Breast Cancer: A Two-Phase Approach
When a breast cancer patient comes to my (Bill's) office, she is usually anxious. She has just had a biopsy, either by needle or by surgery,

and the pathology report is now at hand. The shock is still fresh, and her nerves are on edge. I try to reassure her, if her discovery was early, that her chances of remission are good. In the majority of cases, there is an excellent chance of lasting remission.

When the studies and staging are completed (see chapter 3), it is time to talk about treatment. I explain that treatment involves two phases. They are related, but one does not hinge upon the other. In fact, I tell my patients to imagine a brick wall dividing the two phases of breast cancer treatment. Decisions about treatment in phase one don't necessarily affect decisions about treatment in phase two.

What are these two phases? The first is treatment of the diseased breast so that the cancer will not return there. The second is treatment for the rest of the body, to kill any cancer that might have spread beyond the breast.

Phase One: Treating the Breast

The answer to the question of how to treat the diseased breast depends on the size of the tumor. If the tumor is less than 5 centimeters (approximately 2 inches), the woman usually has two very different options, both of which have good success rates. One is breast conservation surgery, and the other is modified radical mastectomy.

Can I Keep My Breast?

Breast conservation surgery involves removing only the known tumor while leaving the rest of the breast intact. Lymph nodes under the arm are also removed and then the breast receives daily radiation therapy for a period of five to six weeks. This technique has been used for years, but has become particularly popular since 1985, when the scientific literature showed that its survival rate was the same as for traditional mastectomy (removal of the entire breast).

Sometimes breast conservation cannot be done. If a large tumor occurs in a small breast, for instance, removal of the lump means removing nearly all of the breast anyway. Or if the tumor is near the nipple, the nipple must be removed and the appearance is affected. If the cancer is scattered throughout many different breast ducts (this is called multicentric breast cancer), a lumpectomy is not feasible.

There are three distinct facets to breast conservation:

1. The surgeon removes the entire tumor, including a surrounding rim of normal breast tissue. This is called a lumpectomy. Sometimes two or three operations may be required in order to be sure the entire lump has been removed.

2. The surgeon removes the lymph nodes under the arm. This is typically done with a separate incision either at the time of the lumpectomy or at a later date.

3. The remaining parts of the affected breast are treated with radiation. After the wounds have had a chance to heal (which usually takes two to three weeks), radiation is administered on a Monday-through-Friday basis for five to six weeks. This is intended to "sterilize" (kill any residual cancer cells in) the remaining breast tissue.

When Mastectomy Is the Best Choice

Because breast conservation is a multifaceted procedure, it involves the expense of several smaller surgeries and many trips to the radiation center. For the woman who doesn't want to go through all of that, the other option—modified radical mastectomy—is simple and requires just a few days in the hospital to complete. This form of treatment, which has been performed routinely and with great success for several decades, involves removing the entire breast and lymph nodes under the arm in one operation—via one incision. Unlike radical mastectomies, however, it does not involve removing the bulk of the shoulder muscles. The result is less disfiguring and involves less swelling of the arm.

As women become more familiar with the two techniques, more and more will probably choose the conservation method. But a full half of all breast cancers are still treated with mastectomy. The reasons given by women who choose mastectomy are varied, including:

- "My breast just isn't that important to me."

- "Even though I know the risk of the tumor coming back in my irradiated breast is small [see below], I know I wouldn't be able to sleep nights worrying that it could happen to me. It makes me too nervous."

- "My breast has served me well through the years, but now it is simply time to let it go."

- "I would rather have a mastectomy because I know that reconstruction of the breast is possible."

- "Radiation scares me."

- "My husband doesn't care if I have a breast or not."

- "I live a long way from the radiation center, and I don't want to drive each day."

- "I am a working woman, and it is easier for me to take off four or five days for a mastectomy than to come in each day for five or six weeks to take radiation."

Some of these reasons may make sense to you; some may not. The choice between conservation and mastectomy is very sensitive and personal. I urge my patients to do what is best for them, regardless of what others think. There is no right or wrong choice, rather two good options.

You will likely make the best decision after talking to a number of professionals (and you may want to talk to them several times) including a surgeon, a radiation therapist, and a medical oncologist. It will probably also be helpful to talk to women who have had these operations.

I tell my patients that either choice is a good one because each offers a good chance of long-term survival. The possibility of breast cancer returning after mastectomy is virtually nonexistent because the breast is simply not there, while about one in twenty women who have conservative surgery followed by radiation has a recurrence of cancer in the breast. But even in such cases the chances for long-term survival have not been reduced because the new tumor can be removed by mastectomy. This new operation may be discouraging, but in most cases when cancer returns, it is necessary.

What about Reconstructive Surgery?

What can you do for your appearance and self-image after a mastectomy? There are several options. While these are not actually forms of treatment, they are intimately connected with the treatment and the decision-making process preceding treatment.

The first option, and perhaps the simplest, is a breast prosthesis, an artificial breast that is worn inside a mastectomy brassiere. Many prostheses look and feel surprisingly real.

A second option is reconstruction of the breast using surgical techniques. Plastic surgeons use a variety of methods to construct a soft, breastlike mound on the chest after mastectomy. This reconstructed breast does not contain breast ducts, have a natural nipple, or give sexual stimulation to the woman. But it may arouse her mate, will look like a normal breast under clothing, does not have to be worn in a brassiere, and is often cooler than a prosthesis in summertime. A skilled plastic surgeon can produce a reconstructed breast that looks amazingly like the original one.

A plastic surgeon who performs reconstructive surgery of the breast will probably have pamphlets, photos, and perhaps even videos of this procedure. Check them out if you are interested in reconstruction after mastectomy.

Phase Two: Treating the Rest of the Body (Adjuvant Therapy)

Once phase one is completed and the breast is safely treated, your doctor will want to move on to phase two, for breast cancer often involves more than just the breast itself. It can spread through the lymph system or the bloodstream to involve other organs as well.

Adjuvant (literally, "helping" or "auxiliary") therapy is used to fight this spread. This is the treatment used to deal with the question posed in chapter 3—What if the cancer has spread?

How Does Breast Cancer Progress?

Before we look at adjuvant therapy, though, let's look at the five stages through which breast cancer can progress. Then we will better understand the therapies used at each stage. The stages can be compared to the parts of a city neighborhood.

Bill grew up in Minneapolis, where city planners had carefully designed the neighborhoods decades earlier. Each house was on a city block, each block had an alley between the rows of houses, each alley connected to the streets, and the streets connected to highways.

Imagine breast cancer as moving through that neighborhood. It starts out in someone's fenced backyard. The earliest stage of breast cancer (called *in situ*) remains inside that fenced yard. It has a cure rate of nearly 100 percent.

Invasive cancers, on the other hand, have jumped the fence. These have lower rates of cure. Some of them wander up the alleys—analogous to the lymph system, which is slow moving and carries cellular garbage. Others travel the streets—analogous to the blood vessels, which carry faster traffic and provide access to the entire body via the highways (large vessels).

The Five Stages

While no analogy is perfect, and the following stages don't always describe precisely a particular breast cancer, they are helpful to both doctor and patient in predicting the best treatment for each case.

- *in situ* stage. The cancer is still at its site of origin, either the breast duct or the milk-producing lobule.

- Stage 1. The cancer has burst through the walls of the duct or lobule (jumped the fence), but is still small (less than 2 cm. or

¾ inch). Cancers from this point on are called invasive because they have spread beyond their point of origin.

- Stage 2. The cancer has moved down the alley to the lymph nodes, or is larger in size (2 to 5 cm.; or about ¾ to 2 inches).

- Stage 3. The cancer is deeply involved in the lymph nodes or has invaded tissues near the breast, such as muscles or the skin surface. The tumor is most often larger than 5 cm. (2 inches).

- Stage 4. These cancers have traveled the streets and highways of the body to distant sites like the bones, lungs, or liver.

What Is My Risk?

These are the five stages, then, that a breast cancer can move through. The key question for most patients is how far has the cancer spread? That is, has it spread considerably beyond its original point of origin? In medical terms, has micrometastasis (literally, "small change") occurred? Have tiny cancer cells taken root and started to multiply in other parts of the body?

Since oncologists can never know for sure if microscopic spread has occurred, we look at a number risk factors and use a battery of tests to help that prediction. Any or all of the following may be considered in making treatment decisions.

- Tumor size. The larger the tumor, the greater the likelihood that the cancer has spread.

- Age of the patient. This is one situation in which age works to your advantage. Older women tend to have less aggressive cancers than younger women.

- Menopausal status. This may be related to age, but premenopausal women usually have more aggressive tumors than women who have gone through menopause.

- Presence or absence of lymph node spread. Because cancer often spreads through the lymph system, a cancer that has spread to lymph glands is more likely to have also spread to other parts of the body.

- Pathological evaluation. Although the word *pathological* generally means "having to do with disease," in this case it means "under a microscope." Not all breast cancers look alike when viewed through a microscope. When doctors look at cancerous tissue in the pathology lab, they can tell whether it looks "angry" or relatively "docile."

- Presence or absence of hormone receptors on the cancer cells. Hormones can act like keys that turn the "starter switch" of a breast cancer cell, stimulating it to divide and multiply. But the hormones cannot stimulate the cell unless they are fitted into hormone receptors, which act something like keyholes.

    The presence of these hormone receptors on a breast cancer cell is a good sign for two reasons. First, when cancer cells are more aggressive, these receptors are usually absent. Their presence often means that the cancer cells are less dangerous, less likely to spread, and may have a slower growth rate.

    Second, the presence of these receptors means that a relatively simple treatment can be used to destroy cancer cells. Specifically, hormonal therapy can be used with a greater chance of success. Hormonal therapy can be used even in the absence of these hormone receptors, but is more likely to succeed when they are present. We'll explain how this therapy works in a section below.

- Oncogene analysis. As we saw in chapter 1, an oncogene is the part of a chromosome that stimulates abnormal and uncontrolled cell growth. Doctors and scientists are still studying oncogenes as a tool to help predict the risk of cancer's spread. Examination of the oncogenes may help determine if the breast cancer has an "angry" personality and whether additional treatment is needed.

Do I Need Further Treatment?

The doctor will look at all of these risk factors to determine whether the cancer may have moved beyond its point of origin in the breast and whether adjuvant therapy is needed. I usually create a checklist and go over it with my patients. Some indicators are more important than others, such as lymph nodes, tumor size, and presence or absence of hormone receptors. I try to show the patient whether she has all good indicators, all bad, or a mixture of good and bad.

Imagine these two extremes. If the patient is young and has not reached menopause, the tumor is very large, numerous lymph nodes are positive (cancerous), hormone receptors are not present, and the readings from the pathologist are worrisome, most oncologists would say that the chances of the women being cured without adjuvant therapy is only about one in four. Further treatment would be strongly advised and the decision is clear-cut. On the other hand, if the tumor is very small, found only by a mammogram, with negative lymph nodes (no sign of cancer in them), positive hormones (hormone receptors present), in a woman past menopause, and if pathological characteristics are favorable, then the woman has a very good prognosis. She has at least a 90 percent chance of survival at five years, which means that more than 90 percent of women in her situation will be alive five years after the diagnosis—without adjuvant therapy. Doctors will usually not prescribe adjuvant therapy in this situation.

There are two clinical situations in which most oncologists agree that adjuvant therapy is beneficial. The first is that of a postmenopausal woman with positive (cancerous) lymph nodes and the presence of hormone receptors. In this situation, it has been shown that the adjuvant therapy, called hormonal therapy (to be discussed shortly), is called for. In the case of a premenopausal woman with positive lymph nodes, chemotherapy has been clearly shown to be worthwhile.

But sometimes the decision of whether to use adjuvant therapy is very difficult. What if half of the risk indicators are positive and half are negative? In such situations, it is difficult to know whether cancer cells have spread to other parts of the body, and research is not always clear whether further body wide therapy will be beneficial. The question at this point (once the breast has been treated) is whether there are still cancer cells, too tiny for any test to detect, present somewhere in the body.

For this reason the oncologist and patient are faced with hard decisions when risk indicators are mixed. In such situations, I usually draw on the statistics of breast cancer to predict the odds that micrometastasis has occurred. My recommendation to proceed with or to refrain from adjuvant therapy is essentially a best guess based on the information available, the overall health of the patient, and her preference for an aggressive or less aggressive approach.

Clinical Trials

In cases where a doctor is not sure whether to recommend adjuvant therapy, she or he may steer the patient toward a clinical trial. In a clinical trial, a team of cancer researchers, usually at a university, studies situations like these in order to determine which of several treatments is the best. They administer each treatment to a different group of women with breast cancer. Women participating in the trials are usually assigned randomly to the different treatments. Years later, the tests may provide convincing evidence that one treatment is preferred to another.

Clinical trials are used particularly when a certain kind of cancer is being treated by oncologists around the country with widely different treatments, none of which has yet been proven as the best. Of course, there are also cases when no adjuvant therapy is compared with an experimental drug.

If you participate in a clinical trial, you must realize that the chance of being helped is still unknown, but the treatments you receive may well be at the cutting edge of cancer treatment. You will also have the satisfaction of knowing that you may help countless other cancer patients who follow you.

Oncologists refer patients to clinical trials both when it is not clear whether adjuvant therapy is needed and when it is not clear which adjuvant therapy is the best. These trials help advance our knowledge of cancer and its treatment.

What about Chemo?

If you and your doctor decide to go ahead with adjuvant therapy for breast cancer, there are usually two alternatives: chemotherapy and hormonal therapy. The purpose of adjuvant chemotherapy is to rid the body of any microscopic traces of cancer after your treatment for the cancer in the breast. The treatment involves a chemical (drug), and sometimes the chemical used is harsh. There are side effects, but the benefit outweighs them; you have the assurance that you have done everything possible to rid your body of cancer.

Using adjuvant chemotherapy for breast cancer can be likened to using a water hose to put out the final embers of a smoldering campfire. You use the hose because there are some wisps of smoke rising from the ashes. You don't know if the fire will rekindle or not. So, to eliminate lingering doubt, you douse the ashes. The fire may have gone out on its own, but hosing it down makes you feel better—and just may prevent a disaster.

Adjuvant chemotherapy should give you considerable peace of mind because you are using the best technique to eliminate residual traces of cancer. But while hosing down a campfire will certainly put it out, adjuvant chemotherapy is not as foolproof. Unfortunately the odds that chemotherapy will wipe out all the remaining cancer are not 100 percent.

For more information on the drugs and procedures used in chemotherapy and their side effects, see chapter 5.

What about Hormonal Therapy?

The second method commonly used in dealing with suspected microscopic cancer is adjuvant hormonal therapy, used either by itself or in conjunction with chemotherapy.

If chemotherapy is like spraying a campfire with a hose, hormonal therapy can be likened to throwing a wet blanket over the ashes. Just as a wet blanket on smoldering ashes helps keep the fire from coming to life again, hormonal therapy prevents cancer cells from growing. Its effect is less dramatic than chemotherapy, and it needs to be applied over a longer period of time. While chemotherapy is typically used for six months, hormonal therapy is taken for five years or more. In its own way, however, it can be highly effective.

Hormonal therapy works through what could be called cellular trickery. Certain hormones (in this case, estrogen) stimulate cancer cells to grow by fitting into a hormone receptor on the cell—much as a key fits into an automobile's ignition slot and stimulates the engine to start. The most commonly used drug in hormonal therapy, tamoxifen, closely resembles estrogen, so the cell's hormone receptors welcome it eagerly. It fits into the place that estrogen normally occupies. What the cancer cell doesn't know however, is that tamoxifen will shut the cell down, preventing growth. By keeping the real key, estrogen, from fitting into the keyhole, tamoxifen ensures that the cancer cell won't go anywhere. The cancer cell then becomes like a car with the wrong key broken off in the ignition. You can sit down in the front seat, smell the upholstery, put another key up to the slot. But you can't put that second key in, and you cannot get the engine going.

To return to the first analogy, just as the wet blanket must remain on the ashes for a long time to prevent the fire from rekindling, tamoxifen must be taken for a long period of time to prevent cancer cells from growing. The point is to let those deactivated-by-tamoxifen cancer cells decay until they are destroyed by the body's immune system. We can never be certain that all the cells have been destroyed, but researchers estimate that five years of hormonal therapy is sufficient.

Tamoxifen is a powerful tool in the fight against breast cancer and is also being studied as a possible agent in the prevention of breast cancer for high-risk women.

What If It Has Already Spread?

What if breast cancer has already reached stage 3 or stage 4—that is, spread to nearby tissues or distant organs? In stage 3 disease, treatment usually combines chemotherapy, surgery, and radiation. This triple approach incorporates all the treatments we have discussed so far to give the patient the best chance at controlling the disease. Recurrence rates for stage 3 are high, however; relapse by the end of a decade occurs in 70 to 80 percent of patients. For this reason, most oncologists favor an aggressive multimodality approach.

When breast cancer has reached stage 4, sadly, there is no cure. But there is much that can be done to prolong life and make it more comfortable. The right treatment can add months, even years, to a patient's life and reduce the symptoms considerably.

Surgery and radiation have a role in stage 4, especially when cancer has returned primarily to one spot, such as the chest wall or a single bone. Chemotherapy and hormonal therapy are more often used because of their ability to treat the entire body. As we have seen, chemotherapy works faster; hormonal therapy, somewhat slower. Therefore, if a vital organ is imminently threatened, chemotherapy will be favored. If there is no immediate danger and hormone receptors are present, then hormonal therapy, with its milder side effects, is usually preferred. For example, if the cancer has spread from the breast to a rib (which is not immediately life threatening), doctors will usually recommend hormonal therapy, which may take several weeks to produce its effects.

While chemotherapy is generally harsher, the hormonal effects of tamoxifen (the most commonly used hormonal treatment) are also significant. Women complain of skin changes, hot flashes, changes in sexual desire, fluid retention, and sometimes nausea. But by and large, tamoxifen is tolerated well by most patients, and it has proven to be quite effective. Three out of four women whose tumors were originally estrogen receptor positive show a favorable response to tamoxifen.

Then there are women like Gladys, a member of my (Bill's) church, who defies medical explanation. She has been on tamoxifen for nine years under my care, and used the drug for four years with the oncologist who preceded me. Gladys's breast cancer originally spread to her eye, lungs, and bones. But by God's grace and tamoxifen, she is alive and well after thirteen years!

If your cancer is in stage 4, think of Gladys. Hope for remission, pray for healing, and remember that it is not uncommon for a woman at this stage to live for many years.

Another treatment that is being used for advanced breast cancer is bone marrow transplant. It is recommended for younger patients with stage 3 and stage 4 disease, and also for those with multiple cancerous lymph nodes. This procedure involves ordinarily lethal doses of chemotherapy followed by the implantation of healthy marrow a few days later. It is discussed in more detail in chapter 5.

Follow-Up

Most oncologists will want to see patients in remission from breast cancer every four months for a period of two years, followed by six-month visits for the next three years. Mammograms will be needed every year, and perhaps an annual chest X ray. Doctors who prescribe tamoxifen for adjuvant treatment will also recommend an annual pelvic examination because of the very small risk of uterine cancer. The use of blood work and tumor markers varies from doctor to doctor. Bone scans generally are not needed unless there is reason to suspect the cancer has spread to the bones.

Lung Cancer

No discussion of lung cancer should begin without an exhortation to not use tobacco. According to the American Cancer Society, there will be approximately 170,000 new cases of lung cancer in the United States in each of the next several years. As table 1 in chapter 2 indicated, many—perhaps most—of these people would not have lung cancer if they had never smoked or been exposed to someone else's smoking.

There are, of course, instances of lung cancer in people who have never been exposed to tobacco smoke. Nevertheless, few things have been so conclusively linked by cancer research as tobacco and lung cancer. You may possibly get lung cancer if you never smoked. You may escape lung cancer even if you do smoke. But if you smoke, your chances of getting lung cancer are significantly higher than if you do not.

Take a moment to look at the graphs in figure 4, which indicate the changes in the number of cancer deaths from 1930 to 1990. We know from sociological studies that significant tobacco consumption by males preceded that of females by several decades. And these graphs indicate that lung cancer rates for females began to climb markedly several decades after males' rates shot up. In other words, as cigarette smoking increased for each population, so did lung cancer. But the 1990s have also brought us some good news about lung cancer in men. The percentage of American males affected by lung cancer has

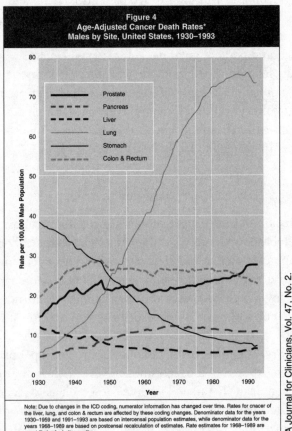

Figure 4
Age-Adjusted Cancer Death Rates*
Males by Site, United States, 1930–1993

Legend:
- Prostate
- Pancreas
- Liver
- Lung
- Stomach
- Colon & Rectum

Rate per 100,000 Male Population

Year

Note: Due to changes in the ICD coding, numerator information has changed over time. Rates for cnacer of the liver, lung, and colon & rectum are affected by these coding changes. Denominator data for the years 1930–1959 and 1991–1993 are based on intercensal population estimates, while denominator data for the years 1968–1989 are based on postcensal recalculation of estimates. Rate estimates for 1968–1989 are most likely of a better quality.

*Rates per 100,000 age-adjusted to the 1970 US standard population.

Data source: Vital Statistics of the United States, 1996.

started to taper off as fewer men light up. If trends persist, we should see a similar decrease among females before too long.

If you have been told that you have lung cancer, one of the first questions you should ask is, "What type do I have?" While there is really only one kind of breast cancer, lung cancer is divided into two broad categories and several subcategories. Each category and sub-category is treated differently. The most important distinction is between small-cell lung cancer and non-small-cell lung cancer.

Small-Cell Carcinoma of the Lung

If your doctor tells you that you have small-cell carcinoma of the lung—or small-cell lung cancer—he or she is reporting to you the lab results from the pathologist who has examined the cells of the cancer tissue under the microscope. While lung cancer can be detected by an X ray or blood test, its precise form cannot be known without a patho-logical analysis of a biopsy. Small-cell cancer of the lung is also called oat-cell carcinoma because its cells are similar in shape to oat seeds lying side by side.

Small-cell carcinoma of the lung occurs in roughly one of every four cases of lung cancer and is completely different from its cousin, non-small-cell carcinoma. The cell's origin is different, its propensity to spread is different, and its responsiveness to chemotherapy is markedly different.

Once your diagnosis is made, you will be asked to go through a variety of tests, the same as for non-small-cell lung cancer: a CAT scan of the lung, bone scan, liver scan, brain scan, liver functions test, and perhaps a bone-marrow biopsy although this is being used less frequently. After administering these staging tests, the oncology team makes an important determination: Is this a limited stage or extensive stage small-cell carcinoma of the lung?

Unlike most other kinds of cancer, small-cell lung carcinoma occurs in only two stages. Limited stage means that the cancer is limited to a relatively small area. The cancer has reached the extensive stage when it has spread to other parts of the body, such as bones, brain, or liver. Determination of the stage enables the doctor to decide on the proper treatment.

Treatment for both stages of small-cell carcinoma centers on chemotherapy. There are two reasons for this:

1. This kind of lung cancer has a remarkable tendency to spread to the bloodstream, even when it exists as just a tiny tumor. Since it spreads so easily and so far, a treatment is needed that can travel to all parts of the body.

2. Chemotherapy is very effective for this particular kind of cancer cell. Researchers are still trying to determine which chemical agent works best, but there are at least a dozen chemicals that help shrink small-cell tumors.

The Limited Stage

The usual treatment for limited-stage small-cell lung cancer is a combination of chemotherapy and radiation to the original tumor site, either during or after the chemotherapy. Some doctors also recommend preventive radiation therapy to the brain. This is because many chemotherapy drugs don't penetrate the brain very well, and the brain could easily become a safe harbor for cancer cells. Radiation therapy, on the other hand, penetrates the brain with ease, and could theoretically take care of escaped cancer cells that the chemotherapy can't reach. We must point out, however, that the value of radiation in this kind of case is debated.

The patient with limited-stage small-cell carcinoma of the lung has grounds for hope. Some studies have reported that as many as 25 percent of patients treated aggressively for this disease will be free of cancer five years later. On the average, though, the life expectancy for someone treated aggressively is one to two years. Untreated, life expectancy is measured in weeks.

The Extensive Stage

The prognosis for extensive-stage small-cell cancer is not nearly as good as that for the more limited form, but the treatment is similar;

chemotherapy is still the treatment of choice. Radiation is not used except when metastatic tumors (those resulting from the spread of the lung cancer) threaten to break a bone or obstruct a vital organ. The average life expectancy for extensive-stage small-cell lung cancer is usually less than one year although some people survive considerably longer. Because of the spread of the cancer, surgery is of little or no help.

As with most cancers, there are still many unanswered questions about the best treatment for this form of lung cancer. Your doctor may suggest that you participate in a clinical trial. These are experimental approaches involving drugs, surgery, radiation, or a combination of these that some researchers believe may offer a better chance of survival. They are offered largely through university cancer centers. (See the preceding section on breast cancer for a full description of clinical trials.)

Follow-Up for Small-Cell Cancers in Remission

If your treatment is completed and your cancer goes into remission, your doctor will probably want to see you now and again. There is no consensus among oncologists about how often these visits should be, but I usually recommend every two to three months and a chest X ray at least two times in the first year. In advanced disease, fewer visits are necessary because the question is usually not whether the cancer will return, but when.

Non-Small-Cell Carcinoma of the Lung

If the pathologist does not see small-cell lung-cancer tissue under the microscope, he or she concludes that the malignancy is probably of the non-small-cell variety. This may sound like an unimaginative name, but for practical purposes the distinction is very useful. Although there are four different kinds of non-small-cell lung cancer, we will discuss them as a group since they tend to be treated in the same way.

To Operate or Not to Operate

Surgery is generally the treatment of choice for non-small-cell varieties of lung cancer. Once it is determined that a patient has this kind of lung cancer, there are two questions to be asked:

1. Is the tumor operable? To answer the first question, the physician usually orders scans (X ray, CAT scan, or nuclear studies) of the bone, liver, and brain to see if the tumor has spread. A chest CAT scan is always performed to determine if malignant lung tissue has moved into adjacent organs or into many lymph glands, particularly those in the center of chest. If it has, surgery may be of little use in treating the cancer. If the cancer is still relatively contained, however, surgery can be quite effective.

   In some cases, there may be anatomical factors that make the tumor inoperable, even if the tumor is small. For instance, the tumor may be on the aorta or attached to the spine and not easily removed. Surgeons in many cancer centers are now using mediastinoscopy (see chapter 3) before surgery. Here, an endoscope is inserted into the space between the lungs to assess the feasibility of successful surgery.

2. Can the patient withstand the rigors of surgery? Sometimes the tumor is operable, but the patient isn't. That is, some bodies are too frail for the trauma of the surgery. The lungs themselves may not be strong enough to withstand removal of any portion. For instance, the same tobacco smoke that has caused cancer in one part of the lung may have damaged the rest of the lung to the point that no portion can be removed without intolerable shortness of breath. Breathing, lung blood circulation, and blood oxygen tests are performed to determine the strength of pulmonary (lung) function. Their results will tell the physician whether the patient will be able to withstand a lobectomy (partial removal of the lung) or even pneumonectomy (removal of an entire lung).

Even if the tumor is deemed inoperable or the patient is not considered a viable surgical candidate, the patient is not abandoned. Radiation can be applied with curative intent. Most oncologists know a few patients who seem to have been cured by this technique when at first all appeared lost.

What Happens after Surgery?

When the surgeon has decided that the tumor is operable and the lung specialist has approved the surgery, surgery is scheduled. This is a major operation that involves opening the chest cavity (thoracotomy). The object is to remove every bit of the tumor; it does no good to remove only part of the tumor.

If the tumor is less than one inch in diameter and has shown no signs of lymph node spread (stage 1), the five-year survival rate is as high as 70 to 80 percent. This means that these patients may have no signs of cancer at the five-year point. With a prognosis this good, there is no need for adjuvant therapy (chemotherapy or radiation).

If the pathologist reports that the tumor is more than one inch in diameter or has spread to lymph nodes, the cancer is in stage 2. The five-year survival rate for this stage of the disease is just under 50 percent. There is no consensus among lung-cancer specialists about whether these patients benefit from adjuvant (auxiliary) chemotherapy or radiation, so you will want to discuss these options with your oncologist, and perhaps consider participating in a clinical trial.

There is no more perplexing group of lung-cancer patients than those in stage 3. This is where the disease has invaded the chest wall, diaphragm, heart surface, or some other important structure between the lungs, such as the esophagus, trachea, or a large blood vessel. Surgery will help some, but not others, at this stage. But even after surgery, residual cancer cells may be left behind in the chest cavity (either because they are so small they cannot be seen or because they are attached to a vital organ like the trachea or aorta). Therefore, radiation therapy is recommended to reduce the likelihood of recurrence.

Historically, only 5 to 10 percent of these stage 3 patients survived after five years. But recently this rate has improved to 25 to 30 percent because of new surgical techniques combined with aggressive use of chemotherapy and radiation. Surgeons are taking out more than in the past because they have developed new methods of rebuilding structures that were once considered impossible to rebuild. As a result more stage 3 patients are surviving after five years than ever before.

Twenty-five to thirty percent may not seem like very good odds to you. But remember, it is much better than what it was just a few years ago. It's a step in the right direction. You will want to discuss with your oncologist which treatment seems best for you, and you may want to be referred to a university for experimental studies. Finally, treatments for lung disease are changing rapidly. By the time you read this book, adjuvant treatment for stage 3 lung cancer may have changed dramatically from what I have just described.

If the Cancer Has Spread Widely

What do you do if your non-small-cell lung cancer has already spread widely from its point of origin? If it has affected other body sites such as the liver, brain, or bone, surgery may be pointless. The prognosis for non-small-cell lung cancer that has spread to other parts of the body (stage 4) is not good; the survival rate after five years is less than 5 percent. Without a miracle, the chances of living even one year are very small.

In these cases, I tell my patients there are three options, none of them particularly attractive:

1. Discontinue treatment, pray for healing, then accept whatever comes.

2. Try chemotherapy for two to three months. Continue it if it seems to work. Discontinue it if it does not. Chemotherapy has a modest track record in non-small-cell lung cancer: It offers a 40 to 50 percent chance of tumor shrinkage. For those patients who are lucky enough to show improvement, life expectancy can increase by six to twelve months. With such odds, the risk from side effects of chemotherapy may be greater than the potential benefit. But the patients whose non-small-cell tumors shrink substantially with chemotherapy think it is well worth the troublesome side effects. Newer drugs now in use include paclitaxel (Taxol), vinorelbine (Navelbine), and gemcitabine (Gemzar). And some of the these newer drugs, particularly paclitaxel, seem

to produce better results; my patients seem to have an easier time with it than with other drugs.

3. Enroll in a clinical trial. As for other cancers, there is almost always a cancer research center trying a new form of surgery, radiation, chemotherapy, or biological treatment. These new therapies may offer a hope that conventional treatments don't. (For more on clinical trials, see the explanation under breast cancer and chapter 5.)

Follow-Up

After completing your treatment, the doctors involved in your care will want to see you return for periodic exams. Typically, they will give you a physical examination plus a chest X ray every three to four months for the first two years, and then every six months or so after that.

At the risk of being overbearing, we want to close this section on the same note with which we began—a word to the wise on tobacco. Smoking is by far the leading cause of lung cancer and, as with most illnesses, an ounce of prevention is worth a pound of cure. We are convinced we would not have had to write these pages on lung cancer if smoking tobacco had never been invented.

Prostate Cancer

In 1993, the American Cancer Society predicted 130,000 new cases of prostate cancer would arise that year. Just four years later, the ACS predicted 210,000 new cases for 1997.

Why the sudden increase in prostate cancer? It is not necessarily due to an epidemic of prostate disease. While our increasingly aging population has produced some new cases, the huge increase was due more to increased screening with PSA (a screening test for prostate cancer) and growing public awareness. Cases that in the past would have gone undiagnosed until a later stage are now caught earlier and counted in an earlier year. The number of prostate cancer cases is significant: They account for 43 percent of all cancers in American males.

Just what is the prostate (not prostrate) gland, and what does it do? The gland is located above the rectum and below the bladder. It encircles the male urethra and manufactures part of the seminal fluid. The incidence of cancer in this part of the body increases with age. Many men who develop this disease will be in relatively little danger because prostate cancer can remain dormant for years. In fact, many men who die at an old age of other causes are found through autopsy to have had prostate cancer.

It is no exaggeration to say that if a man simply lives long enough, he will develop prostate cancer. Another way of saying this is that many men who live a long life will develop prostate cancer but never be aware of it or need treatment for it. The difficult task is to know when the cancer may kill.

Causes

Despite its frequency, we actually know very little about what causes prostate cancer. There has been a suggestion that dietary fat may increase the risk, and there are a few reports of genetic tendencies within certain families to get prostate cancer at a higher frequency and a younger age. In addition, there is an increased risk of prostate cancer in African-American men as compared to Caucasians. The number one risk factor for developing prostate cancer is simply growing old.

What Grade Is It?

There may be no other cancer in men with more riding on its microscopic appearance than prostate cancer. If you have been diagnosed with this disease, therefore, one of the first questions you should ask your doctor is what grade is it?

Prostate tumors are often graded according to their relative aggressiveness as seen under a microscope by a trained pathologist. Assessing the aggressiveness or "angriness" of the tumor helps determine both treatment and prognosis. The grading system most often used is the Gleason's scale, developed by the V.A. Research Group years ago. The Gleason's score ranges from 2 to 10, with 2 being the least angry and

10 the most. A linear relationship exists between the Gleason's number and the chance of spread outside the gland. Gleason's scores of 2 to 4 have a low risk of spread; only 25 percent of them move outside the gland. Gleason's scores of 8 to 10, on the other hand, have a 75 percent chance of spreading beyond the gland.

Has It Spread? How Far?

The second important question to ask is has the cancer spread to other tissues and organs? If it has, how far? The answers will help determine the staging of the disease. (For more on staging and the tests involved to determine it, see chapter 3.) To begin to answer this question, your doctor will order a variety of laboratory tests, including a complete blood count, a set of blood chemistries, and blood enzyme level tests to look for such substances as prostate-specific antigen (PSA). Additional testing is ordered after the physician evaluates the rectal exam, the PSA, and Gleason's score. If the PSA is less than 10, for example, the likelihood of finding an abnormal bone scan is extremely low, so most doctors won't call for one. Some doctors, however, will order it anyway because of the high incidence of arthritic bone disease in older men and because it is useful as a baseline against which to compare future scans. If the PSA is greater than 10, the Gleason's stage is greater than 7, or if the tumor feels large, a bone scan is usually ordered. A CT or MRI scan of the pelvic lymph nodes may also be done in these more worrisome cases to help assess spread outside the prostate gland.

The simplest but perhaps most important test is a physical examination with a gloved finger. By feeling the back of the prostate gland through the rectum, the surgeon (usually a urologist) can get a good sense of how far the cancer has progressed. If the tumor cannot be felt at all, it is in stage A (some would use the classification T1). If it is relatively small, contained within the prostate gland, yet large enough to be felt, it is in stage B (T2). If the tumor extends outside the prostate gland into the fat or seminal vesicles (which help produce and store male semen) next to the gland, it is in stage C (T3). When blood tests or X rays show that the cancer has progressed elsewhere—for instance, past the pelvis and into the lymph glands, blood vessels, or bone—it has entered stage D (T4).

As you can see, it is critical to determine both the grade and the stage of your cancer. If you have a low-grade tumor discovered accidentally at the time of surgery for what was thought to be a benign condition, nothing more may need to be done. All of the cancer may well have been removed by the surgery.

But if, at the other extreme, your tumor is an aggressive one that has reached stage D (T4), you have no chance for a surgical cure. However, much can still be done to relieve your pain and make you more comfortable. We will discuss some of these procedures later.

The greater challenge in choosing treatment involves the in-between stages of B and C (and even some aggressive stage A cancers). After the grade and stage of the tumor has been determined, the next question to ask is should we treat it or sit back and watch? Many factors need to be considered to answer this question. Let me illustrate by introducing Lyman and Fred.

Lyman came to me several years ago with one of those in-between cases. He had recently completed the Virginia Ten Miler, a local long-distance road race, at age seventy-two. Lyman expected life to bring him many more birthdays, so he listened intently as I outlined his treatment options.

Fred, also seventy-two, saw me that same year, but with a different attitude toward life. He had lost his bride of many years, had never had children, and was in poor physical condition. Fred knew, as I did, that he would be lucky to have another birthday. As I reviewed his treatment options, his head nodded up and down quietly as if to say, "That's enough, Doc. Who are we kidding?" He and I agreed that we were better off not doing anything.

Many factors must be considered when deciding between aggressive therapy and watchful waiting: the size of the tumor, the preoperative PSA level, the Gleason's grade, the degree of spread outside the gland, and—most important—the overall health and life expectancy of the patient. Lyman and Fred had tumors of similar grade and stage, but their treatments differed drastically.

As if the decision of whether to treat weren't complicated enough, trying to decide which kind of aggressive treatment to use can also be difficult. Let's consider what is involved.

Getting Aggressive

What is aggressive treatment? Let's first say what it is not. It is not TURP (transurethral resection of the prostate), which is performed thousands of times every month for men all over the country. This is a common surgical technique to relieve urinary problems in older men.

In the process of performing a TURP on a man who has been having prostate symptoms for years, the surgeon may discover a tiny amount of cancer. In such a case, the TURP itself may remove the entire tumor. But this was not the original intent of the surgeon, and this is not the primary purpose of TURP.

Aggressive treatment seeks to kill prostate cancer before it spreads to lymph tissue or the bloodstream. It uses two methods: surgery or radiation, and sometimes both on those cancers that are higher grade (more aggressive) but are still in stages A or B. Sometimes aggressive treatment is used for cases in stage C. Specialists debate whether surgery or radiation is the best choice, but both have enjoyed considerable success; each has similar ten- and fifteen-year survival rates. For many of these patients, there is hope for long-term survival, even cure.

Doesn't it seem as though doctors could have sorted out this important question of treatment options for their patients? It is not for want of trying. The medical literature is full of papers on the topic, but the critical study was thwarted by a lack of acceptability to patients (and their doctors).

A decade ago, one of the U.S. premier cooperative groups (cancer research hospitals that agree to jointly do research) attempted the study. It planned to compare surgery versus radiation for early stage prostate cancer. Sounds good. But in the next two years, not ten patients had been treated and the study closed. It is difficult and scary for doctors and patients to let a "coin toss" determine whether the therapy for prostate cancer will be surgery or radiation; hence few patients entered this important trial. The debate goes on and on. Let's examine both sides.

Surgery

Prostate-cancer surgery (radical prostatectomy) can be performed in one of two ways. One approach involves entering the body in the area between the anus and the scrotum (perineal resection), while the other entails entering above the pubic bone (suprapubic resection). The latter has the advantage of providing the surgeon access to sample or remove the lymph glands, which will help predict if the disease will return.

The advantages of surgery are twofold. First, surgery has the best chance of removing all the disease from the body if the cancer has not spread beyond the initial site. Second, surgery, if the suprapubic approach is used, enables the doctor to better understand how far the cancer has progressed by examining the lymph nodes.

But surgery also has its disadvantages. Some patients will go through this major operation only to have their surgeon discover that the cancer has spread beyond control. Others, especially the elderly and infirm, may risk death on the operating table because of the stress that surgery places on the body. Still others will have the cancer successfully removed but will suffer complications from the surgery itself. For instance, some men will become impotent (unable to achieve an erection). With new nerve-sparing surgical procedures, as many as 50 percent of men who had good sexual potency before surgery will have it afterward.

But if the nonsparing approach is used, only about 10 percent will maintain their sexual potency. This is because the surgeon must generally cut through the delicate nerve systems that control erectile and urinary functions. Yet (and this will be very important for some men) even if the patient is impotent, he may still be able to achieve orgasm and ejaculation; the nerves that control these functions are separate from those that stimulate erection. In any event, if surgery results in impotence, there are therapies now available that can offer surprising help. Ask your urologist about them.

Another problem sometimes encountered after this surgery is urinary dribbling. About 5 percent of patients will develop this. The bladder depends on an intricate network of nerves to allow normal elimination. When these nerves are interrupted, loss of control over the emptying process or closing the urethra can occur. Dribbling can stem from either incomplete emptying or failure to stop the stream.

Radiation

The other option for aggressive treatment for prostate cancers at the A, B, and C stages is radiation therapy. Many doctors and their patients opt for this instead of surgery. Typically, radiation is given as a daily treatment (Monday through Friday, with a weekend rest) over a six- to seven-week period. Most cancer treatment centers use a standard radiation machine (see chapter 5 for more information about the types of machines used). But some centers use brachytherapy, which involves implanting radioactive "seeds" in the patient's prostate gland. These are pellets or ribbons of radioactive metal placed directly into the tumor. Another advance in radiation therapy for prostate cancer is the advent of computerized treatment planning. Radiation oncologists can now use three-dimensional targeting called conformational radiation therapy. In this new approach, a beam of radiation tries to conform to the exact shape of the malignant tumor in the prostate gland. Ask your radiation oncologist for more details.

The advantages of radiation are that it avoids surgery and hospitalization and reduces the risk of nerve damage. Its success rate—that is, its effectiveness in promoting long-term survival—is about the same as that of surgery. It also produces less impotence; only 25 percent of men who were potent before treatment are impotent after treatment.

But radiation also has its disadvantages. It does not provide knowledge, as surgery does, of the extent to which the cancer has spread. The patient also must make many trips to the radiation center over a six- or seven-week period, which can pose a significant problem to those who live far away. Radiation also often produces inflammation of the rectum, bladder, and exposed skin areas.

As many as one-third of patients who receive radiation will still have cancer cells when a biopsy is performed several years later. Although this sounds alarming, some of those tumors may be dormant and not affect the patient's long-term survival.

How should you decide between surgery and radiation? The decision will differ from case to case. Your best course of action is to talk to all the specialists who might be involved in your case. Visit both the urologist (a specialist in the treatment of diseases of the urinary tract, including prostate cancer) and the radiation oncologist to discuss the pros and cons of each option for your particular situation.

As in other cancers, you may be asked to participate in a clinical trial (see a full explanation of clinical trials under breast cancer in this chapter). Your experience with such a trial will help future doctors and their patients decide what is the best therapy for certain kinds of prostate cancer.

In summary, the treatment of in-between prostate cancers is either watchful waiting with frequent doctor visits and PSA blood tests, or aggressive treatment.

Most oncologists operate with the following general rules of thumb. They suggest aggressive treatment if:

- It seems there is a life expectancy of at least ten years.
- The cancer is confined to the prostate gland.
- The PSA is less than 10.
- The Gleason's grade is low to moderate.

Follow-Up
If you and your doctor have decided on aggressive treatment, either surgery or radiation, then you will probably be asked to see your doctor regularly. Typically, patients will return every six months for a period of at least five years to determine PSA levels. A rectal exam is done yearly. For those men who opt for the wait and see approach, a prostate examination and PSA test twice a year and an annual prostate biopsy is typical.

Treatment for Stage D (T4) Prostate Cancers

Unfortunately, stage D (T4) cancer, where the cancer has left the prostate gland tissue and entered the bloodstream or lymph system, is not medically curable. That's the bad news. But the good news is that there is treatment available that can relieve painful symptoms for months to years. For instance, a simple form of hormone therapy can give prompt relief to patients who may have been suffering for months. Hormonal manipulation lowers the level of blood testosterone, a male hormone that stimulates the growth of prostate cancer cells.

Please note that some men in stage D go for years without problems. I have been following a man now for eight years with PSAs that have slowly risen from 50 to more than 250. Despite this rise, he has never had painful symptoms, and so far no treatment has been necessary.

When treatment becomes necessary, there are several different methods of lowering testosterone levels. One method that has been used for decades is surgical removal of the testicles (bilateral orchiectomy). This relatively simple operation, which significantly reduces the level of the male hormone, is relatively inexpensive when compared to medications, and it avoids the danger of forgetting to take your medicine. But, for obvious cosmetic and psychological reasons, relatively few men choose this route.

Another method of lowering testosterone is to use a form of estrogen, a female hormone, which deactivates the prostate cancer cells by counteracting the testosterone. This is usually administered orally in the form of a synthetic estrogen called diethylstilbestrol (DES). Although it is one of the cheapest ways to treat metastatic prostate cancer (prostate cancer that has spread), DES can have serious side effects, including an increased risk of blood clots in the legs and of heart ailments such as heart attacks and heart failure. It can also give men sore and enlarged breasts.

More modern (also higher-priced) techniques lower testosterone levels in the body, either by influencing the testicles (where testosterone is made) or the master (pituitary) gland in the brain. These medications include luprolide and goserelin, which are given by injection and stimulate the production of luteinizing hormone-releasing hormone (LHRH). Like testicle removal and estrogen pills, these provide relief from pain by reducing the amount of testosterone. While at times more expensive, LHRH stimulants have the advantage of a much lower risk of heart problems and blood clots. Hot flashes occur in roughly half the men using these drugs.

A pill called flutamide is an antitestosterone medication that blocks the effect of testosterone without actually lowering the blood levels of the hormone. It is often given in conjunction with one of the therapies already mentioned in an effort to completely block testosterone's influence on the prostate cancer cells. This medication is also quite expensive but has shown promise in the treatment of stage D prostate cancer.

A disadvantage of most of these medications that reduce testosterone or its effects is that they directly affect the male sex drive and the ability to achieve an erection. If this is a problem for you, be sure to talk to your urologist about advances in the treatment of impotence.

As hormone therapy goes on for many months, the prostate cancer cells usually begin to change. They eventually become immune to the effects of hormone manipulation and begin to grow again. Treatment at this point becomes complicated. The patient may need to consider different forms of treatment, including experimental hormones, chemotherapy, or radiation therapy at particularly troublesome spots. Eventually, however, the cancer spreads so widely that the most important goal becomes pain relief. At that point treatment focuses on narcotics, such as morphine, coupled with other pain control techniques. Experimental treatment at a university may be recommended when standard therapies prove ineffective.

On the average, a patient with symptoms of metastatic prostate cancer (stage D), will have a gratifying one- to two-year extension of symptom-free life. For some patients, however, the treatment for metastatic prostate cancer can last for several years. Sometimes, in fact, this cancer becomes more aggravating than life threatening. Because prostate cancer spreads to bone more often than to any other tissue, and because bones are not vital organs, some prostate cancer patients die of something other than their cancer.

What can you do to prolong your survival at stage D? You can try to keep up your body's resistance by consuming a steady supply of nutritious food and by staying as physically active as possible. And try to maintain hope. Remember that some patients with metastatic prostate cancer have maintained useful and meaningful lives for many years. There will be more doctor visits than you imagined, but it is important to keep up with the treatments, pester your doctor for good pain relief, and remember the ones who love and need you.

Colon and Rectal Cancer

Malignancy of the large intestine is one of the most common cancers in the Western Hemisphere.

There will be more than 130,000 new cases in the next year in the United States alone. Recently, there has been a slight dip in the number of cases across the nation. Most experts believe this results from improved public awareness, stool testing for blood loss, and improved diets.

Causes

One of the most striking features of colo-rectal cancer is the preponderance of cases in the industrialized world. Cancers of the colon and rectum are far more common in the West than in Asia or Africa. Some of this may be due to discrepancies in reporting between these regions, but the more likely reason is diet. Saturated fat, which is more prominent in western diets, is thought to be the greatest contributing factor in the onset of these cancers. And a diet with lots of fiber (more common outside the West) is believed to provide some protection against these cancers.

It is a lovely coincidence, by the way, that the same diet (high in fiber and low in fat) that reduces the risk of colon and breast cancer will also help protect us against strokes and heart attacks.

If diet is a factor in these cancers, so is heredity. Cancer of the large intestine can run in families. There is the rare but dramatic Familial Adenomatous Polyposis, a hereditary condition that produces thousands of polyps and almost always leads to colon cancer. And there is the more common case in which a family seems to have more than its share of colon cancers. The genetics of these disorders are being worked out, and genetic testing is being studied for some of the 10 to 15 percent of cases that seem to be inherited. (See the section on breast cancer in this chapter for a closer look at the questions surrounding genetic testing.)

Finally, we know of two diseases of the bowel that are linked to these cancers. Both ulcerative colitis and Crohn's disease raise the risk of colon cancer and need to be watched closely by a gastroenterologist.

A Little Anatomy

In order fully to comprehend the tests and treatments offered for cancers of the intestine, you will need to understand a few points of anatomy. The intestines (also called bowels) are the portions of the food canal that receive partially digested food from the stomach, complete the digestion of that food, and carry the waste products (feces) to an exit from the body (anus).

The longest part of the intestinal tract, which receives food from the stomach and absorbs nutrients, is called the small intestine because it is smaller in diameter than the other part. Cancer is rarely found in the small intestine.

The shorter part of the intestinal tract, which carries waste from the small intestine to the outside of the body, is called the large intestine because of its larger diameter. It is six to seven feet in length and divided into two parts. The higher part is the colon; the lower part, approximately six inches in length, is the rectum.

While the colon is contained within the abdominal sac, called the peritoneum, the rectum is not. Cancers in the rectum, therefore, spread more easily beyond the walls of the bowel and into surrounding lymph glands and blood vessels. Because of this difference, treatment for cancer of one part of the intestine is very different from treatment for cancer in the other. If your doctor tells you that you have intestinal malignancy, you need to ask whether it is cancer of the small bowel or large bowel and, if large bowel, whether it is in the colon or the rectum.

The Polyp

At the center of the best hypothesis we have for the formation of colon cancer, the polyp is a raised area that sometimes appears on the inside lining (mucosa) of the colon. When stool and bile repeatedly pass over it, an irritation is created. This change, over the course of one to three years, may stimulate the formation of a cancer at its tip. As the cancer moves down the stalk of the polyp and into the muscle layers of the mucosa, it becomes dangerous.

Detecting Intestinal Cancer

Blood in the stool heralds the onset of problems. When the passed blood is bright red, this warning is obvious to the patient, but blood can also turn maroon or even black and be missed. An age-old problem regarding cancer, however, is its silent arrival. Intestinal cancer is no different. The blood can be invisible except to stool blood test kits. Hence, cancer of the colon or rectum may originally present with pain, obstruction, or a positive blood test. Whatever leads to the suspicion, further testing will follow.

Now that you have some understanding of the anatomy involved, we can discuss the tests that are used to determine the presence and spread of intestinal cancer. (Most of these tests were explained in some detail in the last chapter, so we won't bother to redefine most of them here.)

The majority of colon and rectal carcinomas are discovered by either endoscopy (a lighted instrument passed into the anus to look directly at the intestines) or X-ray tests (CAT scan or barium enema). These are the best methods of determining specifically where in the bowel the tumor originated.

A wide variety of other tests are used to check for spread of the disease. A CAT scan (and sometimes an MRI scan), for instance, can help check for signs of spread in the lymph nodes or other organs (most commonly, liver and lungs). A chest X ray can detect spread to the lungs, while a rectal ultrasound will show if the tumor has penetrated the bowel wall and spread into adjacent tissues. (See chapter 3 for a full explanation of these tests.)

Then there is an array of blood tests. A complete blood count is often done to look for evidence of blood loss or anemia (early signs of cancer). Blood chemistries and certain tumor markers (see chapter 3) check for spread to the liver, which is a frequent target for cancer spreading from the intestines.

Another valuable test is the one that looks for carcinoembryonic antigen (CEA) in the blood. This blood protein is present in very small amounts in healthy people but in greater amounts in patients who have colon or rectal cancer. Extremely high amounts of CEA may indicate that cancer has spread beyond the bowel.

The Biopsy

Typically, when cancer is suspected, an endoscope is passed through the rectum and a small tissue sample is taken. If a polyp is found with cancer only in its tip and no penetration of the muscle layers, then simply removing it with a heated wire loop is usually sufficient. When cancer is found to have invaded the muscle layers, doctors begin to worry and suggest taking the next step, surgery.

The Surgical Option

Once the tests are completed, treatment begins. Surgery is the most effective treatment for many types of intestinal cancer. The first question, therefore, is usually whether the tumor is operable or inoperable.

An operable cancer is one judged to have a good chance of being cured by surgery—removing every trace of the tumor so that no cancer remains to threaten the patient in the future. Some cancers are considered inoperable but are still treated with surgery. These surgeries are performed not with the expectation of cure, but with the goal of prolonging life and making it more comfortable. For instance, a tumor may be removed from the intestine, even though cancer has spread to other parts of the body, in order to prevent painful obstruction of the bowel.

If the surgeon feels the colon cancer is potentially curable, then a radical surgical resection will be performed. This is a fairly straightforward operation. The surgeon cuts out a segment of the colon (including the tumor), along with a surrounding rim of normal tissue (called the margins) and adjacent lymph nodes. Then the healthy segments of the colon are sewn back together, the wound is closed, and physicians and patient simply wait a day or two for the bowel to start working again.

Surgery for rectal cancer is more difficult for a number of reasons. First there is no covering layer of peritoneum to slow the spread of cancer cells to adjacent tissues, so there is a greater possibility that surrounding tissues will have to be removed. Second, the rectum is deep in the pelvis. It is more difficult to reach than the colon, which is located in the abdominal cavity.

A third difficulty with rectal surgery is that it often involves a colostomy. In the classic operation for rectal cancer (called the abdominal-perineal resection, or APR), the rectum and the muscles of the anal sphincter are removed, which means that the patient no longer has control of defecation (removal of feces from the body via the anus). The colostomy is a procedure that redesigns the large intestine so that feces leave the body through a small hole in the abdominal wall. A colostomy bag, which is an adhesive plastic sac, catches the waste material as it exits.

Newer techniques have enabled some patients to have their rectal tumors removed without a colostomy. Not many rectal cancers are amenable to sphincter-saving surgery (surgery that saves the anal muscles), and not all surgeons know the technique. Generally speaking, only smaller rectal cancers can be considered for this procedure. Ask your surgeon if it can be done in your situation.

Colostomies are not only done for rectal cancers. Some patients undergoing colon cancer removal may require a temporary colostomy. If, for instance, feces present in the intestines at the time of surgery have escaped to contaminate the abdominal cavity, a temporary colostomy will be performed. After several weeks, the bowel segments will be rejoined and the colostomy sewn shut.

A final problem encountered with surgery for rectal cancer is a possible disruption of urinary and sexual functioning. This is because the surgeon may have to cut through a fragile nerve network that affects all of these functions. If the nerves can recover, then return of function is possible, but permanent injury can occur.

Stages of Intestinal Cancer

As for other cancers, the stage of an intestinal cancer must be determined in order to decide which kind of adjuvant (auxiliary) therapy is best. Intestinal cancer is staged according to a number of different systems, but the two most commonly used are the numerical system (1 to 4) and the Duke's system, named after the man who pioneered the staging of colon cancers.

Stage 1 (also called Duke's stage A and B1) is the earliest stage of intestinal cancer. Here the cancer has progressed no farther than the inner layer of the intestine. The cure rate with surgery alone is so high that adjuvant therapy is not needed.

The most advanced stage is stage 4 (Duke's D), where the cancer has spread to distant organs and created tumors there. Unfortunately, there is no known medical cure for intestinal cancer at this stage, so adjuvant therapy is not recommended for these patients either.

Adjuvant therapy is recommended for the in-between stages (stages 2 and 3, or Duke's stages B2, B3, and all Cs). In stage 2 (Duke's B2, B3), the cancer has penetrated the muscular wall of the intestine but not reached the lymph glands just outside the bowel wall. If it has reached those lymph glands, the cancer is at stage 3 (Duke's C).

For stage 1 patients, surgery is in the total treatment. At stage 4, the possibility of cure is remote. If stage 4 spread is limited to just a few deposits in the liver, cure can be gained with the removal of these tumors by a skilled hepatic surgeon. But this is possible for only a small percentage of stage 4 patients; apart from a miracle of God, the vast majority have little or no chance of long-term survival.

We ask most stage 2 and 3 patients to consider the following additional treatments.

Adjuvant Therapy for Colon Cancer

There are two questions to ask in any situation where adjuvant therapy for intestinal cancer is considered. First, are there still cancer cells in the immediate area (sometimes called the tumor bed)? If so, radiation is usually used because radiation is able to focus its cancer-killing energy on a small area. Second, is there a strong chance that cancer cells have spread to distant organs? If so, chemotherapy is the treatment of choice, because it travels throughout the body.

For patients who have had surgery for colon cancer, radiation is not usually recommended for malignancies at stages 2 and 3 for two reasons. Because the colon has the covering layer of peritoneum, there is less risk of spread to the immediate area, and because the colon is fairly mobile in the abdominal cavity, it is hard to pinpoint with radiation.

But there is still a risk that the cancer has spread (metastasized) to other points around the body through the lymph system or bloodstream. Depending on the size of the tumor, the extent of local spread, and the number of local lymph glands already infected with cancer, the risk of micrometastasis (the spread of tiny, invisible cancer cells) ranges from 20 to 80 percent.

Because of these risks, adjuvant chemotherapy for colon cancer is now recommended for some stage 2 colon cancers and nearly all stage 3 patients. The treatment typically combines the use of an older drug called 5-fluorouracil (5-FU) with a newer agent such as leucovorin or levamisole.

The drug 5-fluorouracil works its way into the chromosomes of the cancer cell and helps kill the cancer cell when it attempts to divide. Levamisole is a drug long used by veterinarians to fight intestinal worms in animals; in humans, it seems to empower the immune system to finish off circulating colon cancer cells. Leucovorin is a derivative of a common vitamin; when used with 5-FU, it strengthens the killing power of the drug. The combination of these drugs has reduced the death rate from colon cancers in stage 2 and 3 by as much as a third. Levamisole is taken in a tablet form while 5-FU and leucovorin are given by injection.

Adjuvant Treatment for Rectal Cancer

Because the rectum lacks a peritoneal covering, rectal cancer has a greater chance of recurring near its site of origin. For this reason—and because the abundance of nerves in this area makes a recurring tumor very painful, radiation is often used.

The timing of radiation therapy varies. Some recommend radiation before attempting surgery while others believe radiation therapy should be given after the patient has a chance to heal. Evidence in the medical literature can be found to support both approaches. Your doctor will likely have his or her own preference. In addition, radiation therapy is typically given with an infusion of 5-FU.

Why would chemotherapy be given at the same time as radiation? We will use two analogies to explain the use of this double whammy.

First, imagine you are standing on a lonely wharf at night and see a suspicious-looking character approaching you with his eyes on your pocketbook. If you are forced to fight this character, would you rather fight him when he is sober or when he is stumbling drunk? Of course, you answer, you would rather fight him when he is drunk. So, too, a cancer cell has a harder time surviving the attack of a radiation beam when the cell is already being poisoned by chemotherapy.

The second analogy requires a little knowledge of cellular biology. Cells are most vulnerable to damage when they are dividing. Cancer cells often lie dormant, without growing at all. When they do divide, they do so at random, rather than in a predictable pattern. Now imagine a machine gunner at the bottom of a hill; enemy soldiers are appearing over the top of the hill. If the soldiers crest the hill sporadically, sometimes singly and sometimes in groups, it is difficult for the machine gunner to anticipate them and always be on the alert to fire at the right time. But if they come over the top of a hill in a steady stream, or in a regular pattern, the machine gunner could mow them down more easily.

Radiation therapy also has difficulty killing cancerous cells that divide without a pattern. If radiation is used when the cells are not dividing, it is not as effective. But chemotherapy gets cancer cells to divide in a predictable pattern; radiation then becomes much more effective. It forces the enemy cancer cells to come over the top of the hill at more regular timing, so the radiation machine gun can more easily mow them down.

Despite the use of both weapons in adjuvant treatment for rectal cancer in stages 2 and 3, the outcome is still uncertain. Adjuvant systemic chemotherapy (aimed at the whole body) is known to be effective for colon cancer, and there is growing evidence that the same type of treatment will help patients with rectal cancer. The final decision to use chemotherapy will be made, of course, by you and your doctor and will depend on your health and the stage of your cancer. The question of what is the best form of adjuvant therapy (surgery, radiation, or chemotherapy) is widely debated and still being researched. In order to further this research and try a possibly helpful experimental treatment, you may want to consider a clinical trial. For a discussion of clinical trials, see the section on breast cancer at the beginning of this chapter.

Stage 4 Disease

The prognosis is less ambiguous for those with colon or rectal cancer in stage 4, where tumors have been found in other parts of the body. Outside of the relatively rare situation where a few isolated tumors are found in the liver and can be removed surgically, the standard form of therapy for stage 4 disease is 5-fluorouracil. This drug was discussed earlier in this chapter and is usually used in conjunction with leucovorin, a vitamin-like drug which seems to accentuate the killing power of 5-fluorouracil. It will not cure the patient of cancer, but it may enhance the quality and quantity of the time he or she has left. (We purposely put quality before quantity.) It can shrink metastatic intestinal cancer in a significant number of people, thus easing suffering and sometimes prolonging life.

In a promising new development, scientists have produced a new class of drugs called the camptothecins. These come from the bark of the camptotheca acuminata tree. These new drugs work to disrupt the DNA enzyme topoisomerase-1, which is important to cancer cell reproduction. One analogue derivative is irinotecan (also called CPT-11). It has been newly marketed under the name Camptosar and is available in the United States. It offers a new weapon in the fight against stage 4 disease. It cannot cure the disease and has side effects, such as sometimes severe diarrhea, but it can cause a tumor to regress for a time.

Radiation can also be used for isolated metastatic tumors (tumors that have grown up from a seed cancer cell that has spread), particularly if they are causing pain or obstruction of a vital bodily function. For example, a tumor may be pressing on a kidney or bone. A small amount of radiation can shrink the tumor and allow the patient to live his or her last months in a greater degree of comfort.

Finally, many therapies for all forms of intestinal cancer are still in experimental stages. For example, there are pumps that directly feed chemotherapy into the liver. There are also biological and immunological therapies, and an endless number of new drugs are being tested (see chapter 5 for more on these). Ask your doctor if any of these could benefit you.

Follow-Up

With colon and rectal cancers, your doctor will want to do certain tests after the completion of treatment. For a period of two years, an examination will probably take place every three to four months. This will include blood testing, CBC, chemistries, and a CEA. Some oncologists also recommend yearly chest X rays. Nearly all will ask you to undergo colonoscopy at one year and then every three years or so as long as new polyps are not detected.

Ovarian Cancer

Cancer of the ovary is sneaky. While breast and skin cancers produce tumors you can often see and feel, ovarian cancer is usually invisible and unfelt, buried deep in a woman's pelvis. And tests designed to detect its presence don't always find it. What makes it even more stealthy is that it usually occurs after menopause, when a woman thinks the least about her reproductive organs. Because it is so difficult to detect, nearly three-quarters of all cases are fairly advanced at the time of discovery.

In the United States, more than 25,000 women each year discover they have ovarian cancer.[2] It accounts for 5 percent of all cancers in females and approximately the same proportion of all cancer deaths in women. This makes ovarian cancer the fifth leading cause of female cancer death after cancers of the lung (25 percent), breast (17 percent), colon (10 percent), and pancreas (5 percent). While ovarian cancer does not get the headlines breast cancer does, it is nevertheless a significant threat to women.

Causes

Like many cancers, cancer of the ovary is linked to both heredity and environment. A small minority of ovarian cancers (5 to 10 percent) are the result of known genetic defects. These show up in clusters within a family and usually arise earlier in life than noninherited ovarian cancers. The defective gene BRCA-1 (an oncogene; see chapter 1), which is strongly connected to ovarian and breast cancer, is present in 5 percent of ovarian cancers in women under age forty but in only 1 or 2 percent of cases in women fifty to seventy years old, when ovarian cancer is more common.

Most ovarian cancers are not the result of inherited gene defects, so they do not run in the family. They are the result of either environmental factors or random mutations in genetic material. Environmental factors that have been linked to ovarian cancers include fatty diets, exposure to ionizing radiation (see chapter 2), and few or no pregnancies.

What does pregnancy have to do with ovarian cancer? Researchers think it is related to the monthly cycle in which the ovaries are subjected to rupture (by releasing an egg) and repair roughly every 28 days. One theory is that an ovary that continues this relentless monthly cycle without the built-in rest provided by a pregnancy is more likely to break down and develop malignant cells. But those women who have fewer egg releases because of pregnancies or the use of birth-control pills tend to have less risk of ovarian cancer.

Symptoms and Tests

The most common symptoms of ovarian cancer are pain in the abdomen or pelvis, a change in clothing size (especially at the waistline), and pain during sexual intercourse. Pelvic examination in these cases may find a mass or fluid in the abdomen.

If your doctor thinks you have ovarian cancer, he or she will probably order one or more of the following tests:

- Pelvic examination, in which the doctor feels the vagina, pelvis and rectum for swelling or lumps

- Blood tests that look for CA-125, Beta HCG, and alpha fetoprotein, which are tumor markers (see chapter 3)

- Paracentesis (withdrawal of fluid by needle), especially if there is fluid in the abdomen

- Chest X ray, CAT scan, or MRI of the abdomen and pelvis

- Endoscopy of the colon; or barium enema (for a clear look at the lower portion of the colon)

Choosing a Surgeon

With ovarian cancer, surgery is almost always needed. It enables the oncologist to properly diagnose the cancer, determine its stage (see chapter 3), and begin to eliminate the cancer.

Most obstetricians and general surgeons can remove benign ovaries and perform hysterectomies for reasons other than cancer. But not all of these people have the training or experience necessary for ovarian cancer surgery.

It is particularly important, then, to consult with a gynecological oncologist, a doctor who specializes in cancers of the female reproductive system and is experienced with this kind of surgery. This physician does not have to do your surgery, but his or her advice should be sought at least to confirm the diagnosis or as a second opinion.

The Surgery

While the surgeon and patient are still in the operating room, a preliminary diagnosis can usually be made. If the tumor is benign, it alone will be removed (especially if the woman wants to remain fertile). When cancer is found, the surgeon will need to remove much more tissue and perform a radical hysterectomy.

This surgery is extensive. The surgeon will make a large vertical incision to explore the whole abdomen and pelvis, wash those cavities with a saline solution to flush out cancer cells, and remove the tumor without rupturing it if possible. In addition, he or she will perform a total abdominal hysterectomy (removal of the uterus), a bilateral salpingo-oophorectomy (removal of the ovaries and fallopian tubes), and an omentectomy (removal of the omentum—a layer of fat in the abdomen—and some pelvic and abdominal lymph nodes). Finally, the surgeon will take random samples of tissue from the abdominal cavity, all the way up to the diaphragm muscles just under the lungs, to look for further evidence of cancer.

As you can see, this is a huge surgery. But experienced surgeons can perform this quite successfully and in the process remove all "bulky" disease, that is, all clumps of cancerous tissue—up to a point. If cancer is not attached to an organ, it will be removed completely. But if it is growing on an organ, such as the bladder or liver, the surgeon will need to leave behind a tiny layer of cancer to avoid puncturing the organ while trying to peel off the cancer.

If the cancerous tumor is growing on or around the intestines, however, surgeons will typically remove the section of the bowel—tumor included—and attach the two remaining segments of the intestine together. The goal is to cut away as much of the cancer as possible, leaving no more than 1 to 2 centimeters (approximately ¼ to ½ inch). In medicalese, this is called "debulking" surgery.

Pathology and Staging

After surgery your doctor will consult with the pathologist and the surgeon to determine what further treatment is needed. The pathologist who examined the tissues taken from your abdomen will tell your doctor what kind of tumor you had. For 90 percent of women with ovarian cancer, the tumor arises from the lining of the ovary (the epithelium). The other 10 percent of ovarian cancers come from the middle of the ovary, where the eggs are made. In rare instances, the tumor is said to have low malignant potential. Such cells look like they could go either way—benign or malignant. Women with tumors of low malignant potential don't have ovarian cancer but need to be watched closely.

The surgeon who explored your peritoneal cavity (peritoneum is the smooth transparent membrane that lines the cavity of the abdomen) from the dome of the abdomen just under the lungs all the way down to the floor of the pelvis, will determine what stage your cancer is. If the cancer is limited to your ovaries, it is stage 1; if it has invaded the pelvis, it is stage 2. Stage 3 cancer has migrated outside the pelvis and into the abdomen. In stage 4 the cancer has spread to distant parts of the body.

With the combination of information from pathology and staging, a prognosis can be determined. If the pathologist finds that your tumor was malignant but at a low grade (or aggressiveness), and the surgeon indicates that it is in a low stage (has not traveled beyond the ovary), the chance of recurrence of the cancer may be small and no additional therapy may be recommended. But if the cancer looks angry under the microscope (high grade), or if cancer cells are found outside the ovaries (particularly if they are found in other places in the abdomen), further treatment will be recommended.

Chemotherapy

Some Canadian research hospitals prefer to give radiation to the whole abdomen of high-risk women (whose cancer was more advanced) after surgery. In America, on the other hand, the treatment of choice is chemotherapy. The goal for each kind of therapy is to eradicate stray cancer cells in the abdomen and pelvis and avoid recurrence in the future. Both kinds of treatment have merit; most women in America will undergo several cycles of chemotherapy.

For decades, patients with ovarian cancer have received chemotherapy. But in the last few years oncologists have discovered a drug combination that is more effective than ever. It delivers a one-two punch, using both a platinum-based drug and paclitaxel (also known as Taxol). The most commonly used drugs derived from platinum are Cisplatin and Carboplatin. Taxol is an extract from the Western Yew tree.

Six cycles of these drugs are usually given, and each is administered intravenously. A cycle equals one session, which lasts several hours. Cycles are administered every three to four weeks. The drugs may be given by your surgeon or medical oncologist, either in a doctor's office or in a hospital room (because of the long infusion times, some doctors' offices are not equipped to handle this form of chemotherapy).

The side effects of these drugs include nausea, hair loss, tiredness, low blood counts, and an increased risk of infection. Blood transfusions may be needed if blood counts drop too low. These side effects are burdensome, but most patients conclude they are worth bearing because they significantly increase the chances of long-term survival and even cure.

So don't despair, dear patient! Chemotherapy is not pleasant, but it can make the difference for many with advanced cancer. Because surgery leaves behind tiny deposits of cancer, your chances of long-term survival go up markedly with chemotherapy, which tries to kill these tiny deposits.

Other Issues

For years doctors have been putting chemotherapy drugs directly into the abdominal cavity rather than injecting them through the veins. This is called intraperitoneal chemotherapy. Theoretically, this option would appear to be more effective because it applies these effective drugs directly to cancerous tissue. But in practice it has not yet been proven to be significantly better than intravenous chemotherapy. And it is more difficult to administer.

Also of some controversy is second-look surgery—performed some months after the first surgery in order to reexplore the abdomen after all adjuvant therapy (chemotherapy or radiation) has been completed. In the past, this second surgery was performed for several reasons. It was considered necessary to predict the woman's chances of relapse and was an opportunity to remove any residual cancer remaining after adjuvant therapy was completed. If additional cancer was found, then more or different chemotherapy was used. But if no cancer was found, both patient and doctor could feel more assured that medication was no longer needed.

At one time second-look surgery was standard procedure. But most oncologists no longer recommend it so routinely. First, it is a difficult surgery to endure since it reopens the skin and abdominal muscles, which means longer recovery time. Second, studies have not proven that the survival and cure rates of women who underwent this second surgery were significantly better than those of women who did not. Therefore many now argue that intraperitoneal chemotherapy and second-look surgery should be performed only in the setting of clinical trials, where researchers can better study its effectiveness.

There Is Hope!

I said at the beginning of this section that ovarian cancer is sneaky. I also want to add that it is curable! Although it is deceptive in appearance and can be terrifying if left untreated, through experienced and aggressive treatment, ovarian cancer can be conquered.

When ovarian cancer has spread throughout the abdominal cavity, the chance of survival five years after chemotherapy ranges from 30 to 70 percent. For women whose cancer has not penetrated outside the ovary, the survival and cure rates are far higher. But even when the cancer has traveled beyond the abdomen to some distant site, 10 percent of women who have been treated will be alive after five years.

One of the most enjoyable parts of my day is when I see patients who are no longer undergoing chemotherapy. They have the spring back in their step, and all their hair on their head. I have treated many women with ovarian cancer who are years past chemotherapy and are leading active, healthy lives. This includes some whose ovarian cancer was advanced.

Remember that statistics are only statistics. I remind my patients that when someone cites an 80 percent cure rate for a malignancy, for example, this applies only to a group, not an individual. The person sitting in an examination room with her doctor will never be 80 percent cured; she will either be 100 percent cured or 0 percent cured.

I ask my patients, "Which one should we shoot for?" The point I want them to understand is that despite odds that may be less than 100 percent, our goal will be to cure. I also remind them that while we can aim for physical cure, only the Lord can provide a spiritual cure. He offers eternal life and joy with him in the midst of suffering. We'll look more carefully at what this means in chapters 9 through 13.

Follow-Up

After you have finished your treatment, you will have to sit down with your doctor to discuss what comes next. He or she will probably recommend what researchers have advised: For the first year you should visit the doctor every three months, every four months for the second year, and then twice yearly until you reach the five-year mark. At these visits blood work will be done to check for (among other things) the tumor marker CA-125 (see chapter 3). In higher-risk women (whose cancer was more advanced), doctors may also order chest X rays and CAT scans.

Insurance plans and physicians' experience differ slightly from state to state and country to country, so don't be surprised if your schedule varies from these guidelines. They are just that—guidelines not rules.

During this recovery period, most women find that their worries and anxieties diminish with each passing month, especially as their hair begins to grow back. I advise my patients that the best way to strengthen that recovery is to maintain an active prayer life, regularly asking God for his continued blessings of healing, strength, and peace.

Skin Cancer: Melanoma

Our skin is our protection from the world. It shields our organs and all the other inner workings of the body from hostile agents in the outside world. We need every square inch of it. But we don't need skin cancer.

Cancers of the skin come in all shapes, sizes, and colors. Most can be recognized by someone who knows what to look for, but some are more difficult to detect. Ask dermatologists who have a bit of gray hair, and they will tell you that for every two or three skin cancers they can easily detect in an office visit, one will fool them if they are not careful. This makes them nervous, and it ought to make us nervous when we see new or irregular spots on our skin. If you suspect skin cancer is a danger for you or your loved ones, please study what follows.

Of all the tumors of the skin, melanoma is the most dangerous. It alone arises from pigment-producing cells (melanocytes; both melanoma and melanocytes come from the Greek word for "black") and so behaves very differently from the more common skin cancers, basal cell carcinomas and squamous (from the Greek word for "scaly") cell carcinomas. Because these common skin cancers do not inflict much harm and can be treated by removal alone, this chapter will focus on the more dangerous melanoma.[3]

The Bad News: Rising Risk

Melanoma is becoming a public health issue, both in the United States and abroad, because of its alarming rate of increase. The American Cancer Society notes that melanoma currently accounts for 3 percent of all invasive cancers (they invade healthy tissue) in men and women. It is estimated that in 1997, for example, there will be 40,000 cases of malignant melanoma in the United States, resulting in 7,000 deaths.

Melanoma is spreading at an astonishing rate. According to the Melanoma Cooperative Group at New York University, the average American citizen in 1930 had a 1 in 1,500 chance of developing malignant melanoma. By the 1980s, that risk had jumped by a factor of ten, to 1 in 150. By 1996, less than a decade later (!), the risk had jumped again to 1 in 87.[4] Some experts believe that these rates will continue to rise, making melanoma a potential epidemic in certain parts of the world. Those most at risk are Caucasians living near the equator, especially in Australia, Israel, Hawaii, and the desert regions of the United States.

The Good News: It Is Preventable and Curable

Rates are soaring, but they don't have to. And treatment is better than ever. That's the good news. Better kinds of treatments have dramatically improved five-year survival rates in the last few decades. Public awareness of the disease is also growing, which should promote both early detection and prevention (by avoiding the sun and using sunblocks).

Melanoma is easier to detect than some other cancers because the vast majority occur on the face, extremities, back, and shoulders. Yet sometimes these cancers are located in unusual places. I once saw a young woman who had difficulty swallowing. When our team was looking for the cause of the problem, we discovered a malignant melanoma in her esophagus that was caused by a melanocyte somewhere in the lining of her digestive tract. So while melanomas are usually much easier to find than many other cancers, do not overlook any new and unusual development in your body. Let your doctor know if you notice something.

Causes

There is little doubt that the principal cause of melanomas is ultraviolet light. To help us understand ultraviolet light, let's try to recall a little high school science. The light visible to the human eye includes a wide spectrum of color, from red to violet, ranging along the following pattern: red-orange-yellow-green-blue-indigo-violet. We see this spectrum in a rainbow or when we hold a prism up to the light.

On either side of the spectrum are other kinds of light that we can feel but not see. The best example of longer wavelength light is the light to the left, or below, red called infrared (infra means "below"). This is a form of heat and is used in restaurants to keep food warm. To the right, or above, violet is shorter wavelength light called ultraviolet (ultra means "above"). This light contains high energy waves that can damage genetic material.

If you hang around the swimming pool or local tanning center long enough, you will expose yourself to dangerous levels of ultraviolet rays.

You risk causing cancerous changes to your skin, producing basal cell and squamous cell carcinomas or the far more perilous melanomas.

These two basic types of skin cancer are caused by different kinds of sun exposure. Basal cell and squamous cell cancers are usually caused by chronic (long-term) exposure to sunlight or another source of ultraviolet rays. Melanomas, on the other hand, are generally triggered by higher doses of intermittent sunshine. So the most dangerous activity of all is for a light-skinned person who typically stays indoors to take a week off for a sun feast and get a blistering burn. Burns that produce blisters, especially in childhood, are strongly linked to melanoma in adults.

Sometimes I startle church and civic groups by telling them that letting our children get severe, blistering burns is a form of child abuse. Most of us would not hesitate to call the local social services if we saw a child with cigarette burns on her skin, but many of us continue to overlook the importance of sunblocks and other sunburn prevention measures when our children play outdoors all summer long. One of the most important things we can do as parents is to care diligently for our children's skin at this stage in their lives by providing sunblocks and appropriate clothing.

Other Risk Factors

There are some other risk factors that we cannot control but should be aware of:

- Fair-skinned, nontanning Caucasians are more likely to get melanoma.

- Males are at higher risk than females.

- Atypical moles (or dysplastic nevi, as doctors like to call them) are more susceptible to melanoma. These moles have irregular shapes and are often spotty in their brown coloration. Be particularly careful if you have many of these irregular moles and there has been melanoma in your family: You may have a genetic predisposition to this disease. Members of families with the

Dysplastic Nevus Syndrome (also called FAMM, or "familial atypical mole/melanoma syndrome") can have an 80 percent lifetime risk of developing a melanoma.

- Giant congenital nevi also raise risk. These are generally 5 to 7.5 centimeters (2 to 3 inches) in diameter, deeply brown, raised moles that develop early in infancy and childhood. In time they may develop into melanoma. Be sure to get them checked regularly and to avoid sunburn.

Diagnosis

As melanoma rates have mushroomed in this country, public health programs have made efforts to tell us how to distinguish troublesome from harmless moles. We should be ever vigilant if our loved ones have many or what appear to be risky moles.

What are the worrisome features to look for? The following four are the most important:

- Change in shape of an old mole, particularly when it becomes asymmetrical or develops an irregular border.

- Any change in color or pattern of color.

- Change in diameter of an old lesion.

- The development of pain, bleeding, itching, or ulceration on or around a mole.

If one or more of these factors is present, your doctor will decide whether a biopsy (a tissue sample) should be taken. The decision will depend on the number and severity of the above factors.

Biopsies can be taken by a nurse practitioner, physician's assistant, family doctor, general surgeon, dermatologist, or another specialist. One caution should be mentioned, however: If melanoma is suspected, shave biopsies (very thin samples), cryosurgery (freezing), and electrodesiccation (heat) are not sufficient. They do not provide tissue samples that are large enough or of good enough quality to give pathologists all the information they need for an accurate diagnosis.

Most experienced clinicians use a technique that removes the whole mole plus 1 to 2 millimeters (about 1/16 of an inch) of tissue around the mole. If the mole is benign, then it is gone for good and cannot become cancerous. But if it is malignant, and a melanoma as well, more surgery will be needed.

Types of Melanoma

There are four types of melanoma.

1. Superficial spreading melanoma. This is the most common melanoma; it accounts for 70 percent of all cases. This kind is flatter than it is tall. While it includes a variety of pigments within its borders, the most common is bluish-black. But red and white lesions are also seen.

2. Nodular melanoma. This is the easiest to detect because it "pops up" quite suddenly, either out of what seems to be thin air or a pre-existing mole. It is usually dark blue-black and accounts for 10 to 15 percent of all melanoma cases.

3. Lentigo maligna melanoma. These melanomas, which make up 10 percent of all cases, develop from noncancerous lentigo malignas, which are wide, flat, and wandering light brown spots on the face or neck. These noncancerous brown patches can be present for decades before they develop into melanomas, so it is very important to get these patches regularly checked by a doctor.

4. Acral lentiginous melanoma. These deeply pigmented moles are fairly uncommon (only 2 to 5 percent of melanomas), but should not be overlooked for two reasons. First, they are found in places we would not suspect: at the ends of the fingers and toes and sometimes under the nail. Second, members of highly pigmented races get these melanomas at much higher rates than Caucasians; in fact, 50 to 90 percent of all melanomas in blacks, Hispanics, and Asians are acral lentiginous melanomas.

Staging

When pathologists get a tumor biopsy, they look for a number of things to determine how far the cancer has progressed. Indicators include how far it has penetrated the skin, how many dividing melanoma cells they can see, whether they find small break-away tumor deposits outside the tumor itself, and most important, how high or thick the melanoma is after it has been removed.

Pathologists use two different methods to measure the size and seriousness of a melanoma tumor. The first, called Clark's levels, indicates the degree of invasion into the skin and determines the risk of spread. The least invasive lesions are at level 1, and the most invasive are at level 5, which means the melanoma has penetrated deep into the fat beneath the skin.

The second method, called Breslow's levels, measures the height of the melanoma in millimeters. This helps predict the patient's prognosis. For example, when the melanoma is less than three-quarters of a millimeter thick, the five-year survival rate is more than 90 percent. With each millimeter of added thickness, the five-year survival rate falls. If draining lymph nodes (those close to the tumor) are also positive (cancerous), then survival rates drop further.

As in most other cancers, the presence of cancer beyond the lymph nodes means the cancer has reached the highest stage, and the five-year survival rate is near zero. I tell patients at this stage that their melanoma is in God's hands, and the purpose of therapy is to make them comfortable or help us learn more about the disease if they choose to participate in experimental therapy.

Surgery

As for any cancer, it is important that your surgeon be someone who is familiar with the specific cancer and has treated the disease regularly. Surgical treatment for melanoma continually evolves as research shows us more effective ways to deal with it; you will feel more confident if you know that your surgeon is not handling melanoma for the first time.

One change in the treatment of this disease over the years is the amount of surrounding tissue cut out. At one time 5 to 7.5 centimeter (2 to 3 inch) margins around melanomas were routinely removed by surgeons. But research has demonstrated that much less needs to be excised; the amount depends on the Breslow's stage (the height or thickness of the lesion). Most lesions require a rim of only 1 to 2 centimeters (⅜ to ¾ of an inch) of tissue to be removed, as long as the edge of the incision is negative (completely free of cancer) when looked at through the microscope.

The importance of this negative margin cannot be overstated. While the cosmetic appearance of the wound is important, it should never compromise the necessity of removing all cancerous tissue. There must be a rim of normal tissue all the way around the tissue that is cut away. In most cases this allows for a scar that is not unsightly. But if a large section of tissue is removed, particularly in visible areas, plastic surgery and skin grafting may be necessary.

One decision your surgeon will make is whether to also remove lymph nodes, and if they are removed, which nodes to take out. If the melanoma is on a leg or arm, the lymph nodes affected would be in the armpit or groin of the same side. If those nodes do not feel enlarged (doctors often use their fingertips to determine this), and the Breslow depth is less than one millimeter, then lymph nodes are usually not removed.

If the lesion is on the trunk of the body or is more than one millimeter thick, it is more difficult to decide what to do. Some surgeons will leave the lymph nodes alone because research has not shown conclusively that removing them improves survival rates. Others will try to determine which nodes are probably affected using a method called sentinel node mapping. This method (also called scintigraphy) determines which node would likely be the first affected. The surgeon then checks that node to see if the cancer has spread into the lymph system (just as a sentinel on watch in wartime will call out an alarm if he sees danger coming). Because lymph node removal is still controversial, you should discuss the pros and cons of this procedure with your oncologist or inquire at the melanoma clinic in a university hospital.

Adjuvant Therapy

If your lesion was shallow—less than one millimeter—treatment after surgery may be limited to careful reexamination of the original scar as well as nearby lymph nodes and the entire skin. Lifelong follow-up is essential to protect against recurrence. Be careful to use sunblocks and avoid sunburn.

If your lesion was more than one millimeter thick, the chance of its spreading to the rest of your body is greater. This is why researchers and physicians continue to diligently search for ways to treat the whole body, not just the area from which cancer was removed. Traditional chemotherapy has a poor track record with melanomas. While not entirely useless, it rarely cures, has significant side effects, and in advanced cases reverses the cancer only 10 to 25 percent of the time.

For these reasons melanoma researchers are experimenting with biological therapy—the use of substances that our bodies already make—to attack cancers. For some time scientists have suspected that melanoma is influenced by the patient's immune system. Hence research has focused in recent years on substances like interferons and interleukins, which are proteins made by the body to activate our immune systems. Ask your medical oncologist (who specializes in chemotherapy) if interferons or interleukins would be appropriate in your case.

If your disease is in an advanced stage and has traveled to other parts of your body, treatment is usually palliative, that is, directed to making you feel comfortable, with little or no hope of cure. But don't give up hope. Experimental therapies are offered at melanoma centers (usually located at university hospitals); one of these may one day provide long-term survival even in advanced cases. And in the meantime, melanoma is notoriously unpredictable. Some people with very advanced melanomas nevertheless survive for years. That "some" may include you.

Two years ago Evans walked into my (Bill's) Lexington, Virginia, office with the bad news in his hands. He was carrying the biopsy reports from a local university hospital indicating that the spot on his lung was cancer, which had spread from a shoulder melanoma that had been removed three years before. The university doctor had advised him to start chemotherapy. But after we talked it over, neither of us was too keen about doing that. Evans simply didn't feel bad yet, and chemo was likely to change that. So he didn't do what his university doctor prescribed.

At this writing it has been two years since that decision, and Evans still has not taken any chemotherapy. Instead, he and his wife, their families, and all their friends—plus their churches and their friends' churches—have been praying. Today his chest X ray looks normal, he is free of cancer symptoms, and his confidence that Jesus will call him home when things are ready is at an all-time high.

As with any advanced cancer, a sense of hopelessness can be overcome by appealing to the source of all hope—the living God. He can do what doctors cannot.

We have just visited six common cancers in North America—their eradication would eliminate over half of all invasive cancers. If the cancer of concern in your life isn't one of these, thank you for taking the time to read this long chapter. We hope it adds new insight into the concepts of stage, prognosis, treatment decisions, and experimental therapy. We also hope it gives you a strong sense that cancers are usually best treated when found early. Even in advanced cases, however, much can be done.

5

What Can You Do for Me, Doc?

---

*Surgery, Radiation, Chemotherapy,
and Biological Treatments*

Earlier we compared the cancer patient's experience to that of running a race in which hurdles must be jumped on the way to the finish line. The first hurdle to overcome is the initial shock of the cancer diagnosis while the second is going through various tests to determine if and where the cancer has spread. The next hurdle, possibly the most burdensome, is to go through treatment.

I (Bill) used to be surprised by how the different kinds of treatments seemed to blur together in my patients' minds when I first discussed therapy options with them. Words like surgery, biopsy, cobalt, chemo, and X-ray treatment often seemed confusing to patients. But after a while, I realized that I should not have been surprised. After all, I went to school for nine years after college to study medicine. And I was not facing a possible threat to my life when I was learning these things. Why should I have been surprised when my patients didn't clearly understand therapy after a one-hour session in my office?

This is precisely why we have written this book in general and this chapter in particular. It explains in clear, simple language what each of the major cancer treatments involves, the purpose of each treatment, the indications for its use, and the possible drawbacks. Reading the chapter and then referring back to it when needed later should help dispel most or all of the confusion that arises in discussing the various treatment possibilities.

Although the details of treatment are sometimes complex, there are really only four types of treatment for cancer: surgery, radiation, chemotherapy, and biological (or natural) therapy. We have already looked at most of these to some extent in previous chapters in connection with specific kinds of cancer. In this chapter, we will focus on these treatments in a little more detail and also review some considerations in working with your doctor.

Heal with Steel: The Option of Surgery

When discussing the various forms of cancer treatments, we find that it helps to use a garden analogy. If you think of the body as a healthy garden and cancer cells as weeds, you can get a clearer picture of the task of treatment at various stages of the disease.

If, for example, a weed or group of weeds is confined to one corner of the garden, the gardener's job is not too hard. The one unsightly patch can be removed without damaging the good plants in the rest of the garden. After that, the gardener may need to sterilize the soil or mulch the garden to prevent future weeds, but the simple weeding probably took care of the problem.

If the weeds are spread throughout a garden, however, the gardener knows the job ahead will be tough. The gardener can try to wade in and dig up each weed one by one but in doing so will run the risk of trampling the healthy plants, and some may die as a result. If the garden has been neglected too long, it may be too late to save it.

So, too, if cancer is isolated in one part of the body, the surgeon can remove it. The patient may then be permanently cured. In some cases the patient may need additional therapy (adjuvant treatment) such as chemotherapy or radiation after the surgery. If the cancer has spread to different organs in the body, however, the picture is very different, and surgery may be useless. The surgeon could remove the cancer from one or even two spots; but what good would that do if the cancer is in ten other locations as well?

Does Surgery Spread Cancer?

I have found that surgical removal is the easiest treatment for my patients to understand. It takes very little effort to convince most people that this is a valid form of treatment. Cancer is the specialty of some surgeons; these physicians are called surgical oncologists. Others — general surgeons, thoracic (chest) surgeons, and plastic surgeons — still do most of the surgery for cancer in this country and others. But true surgical oncologists have different and longer training, and are still somewhat uncommon.

Some patients are afraid of surgery because they think it will somehow cause their cancer cells to spread. "Once it hits the air," some have told me confidently, "it spreads everywhere." Well-intentioned relatives or neighbors have told them this and made them adamantly opposed to any surgical solution.

If this were true, of course, patients could not be blamed for their refusal to undergo surgery. After all, the threat of cancer spreading is terrifying. But the idea that properly performed surgery makes cancer spread like dandelion seeds blown in the wind is absolutely false — and this particular cancer myth has probably done more harm over the years than any other. Surgery is the key to many cancer cures; without it many patients who otherwise would live will probably die. To stubbornly hold on to this myth, when all the evidence is against it, is both stupid and life threatening.

What about Lasers?

Laser surgery is one new technical advance in cancer surgery that has generated a great deal of interest. Because of its ability to focus intense light on a tiny area, a laser beam can vaporize and cut normal tissue with very little damage to surrounding structures and can thus reduce bleeding, scarring, and pain in many instances. Laser therapy can therefore be invaluable for controlling bleeding, relieving obstructions, and removing certain small cancers—particularly ones that can be reached by endoscopy (see chapter 3). For various reasons, however, laser surgery is not always effective, and it can be expensive. At this point it has not proven to be significantly or consistently better than traditional surgery.

Even though lasers have not replaced scalpels, however, they have proven very beneficial in some situations. It may be worthwhile to ask your physician if a laser is applicable to your situation.

Getting Buzzed: The Option of Radiation

Radiation is another way to kill cancer. If surgery is like pulling weeds from the garden, then radiation is a little like letting the weeds wilt in an overdose of sunshine. (Yes, we know this is not likely in a garden of healthy plants. No analogy is 100 percent accurate.)

Like surgery, radiation works best for tumors confined to one area of the body. While it is possible to irradiate the whole body, such a procedure would probably kill the patient. This, in fact, is precisely what happened to many of the victims of the atomic explosions at Hiroshima and Nagasaki. Their whole bodies were exposed to the radiation from the bomb, and many of them died of radiation sickness. Only in very unusual circumstances (certain cases of prostate cancer and skin lymphoma) is the entire body subjected to radiation.

How Radiation Works

But what is radiation therapy anyway? It is the use of high-energy beams (X rays and gamma rays) that are colorless, odorless, and painless. These beams can be compared to a beam of light from a flashlight, but radiation's "light" is of a very different wavelength. It uses much higher energy and is infinitely more damaging than visible light. If this high-energy beam of radiation is repeatedly focused on a group of cancerous cells, as in a tumor, the cells can often be killed and the tumor eradicated.

Radiation treatments kill cancer cells by damaging DNA (see

chapter 1) and thus preventing the cells from reproducing themselves. Fortunately, normal cells tolerate radiation much better than cancer cells, especially when radiation is applied at low levels over a longer period of time. When radiation is given over several weeks, both cancer cells and normal cells are damaged. But normal cells can usually repair the damage, while cancer cells are unable to reproduce. The hoped-for result is the eventual death of the tumor in a given area.

The Radiation Team

The doctor who directs the application of radiation to a patient is a highly trained specialist who works with a team of other specialists in the radiation center. The team includes nurses, clinical physicists, and radiation-dose specialists who use devices such as computer simulators and scanners. All of these people and devices work together to ensure that radiation is delivered accurately to cancerous tissue with an absolute minimum of scatter to surrounding flesh.

The radiation itself can come from a variety of sources. Since very few substances on earth emit radiation naturally, sources for radiation therapy must be prepared by scientists.

One common source is cobalt. This is a naturally occurring metallic element that is prepared in a way that makes it radioactive. It is then heavily encased in lead—which is resistant to radiation—until it is needed for treatments. The radiation therapist maps out the area of the body that needs treatment, and directs the beam from the radioactive cobalt encased in the machine toward the tumor cells.

More modern machines use a linear accelerator. This is a variation of the atom smashers you may have read about in high school or college. These devices shoot electrons at astounding speeds into an immovable target. At impact, a tiny beam of radiation energy is emitted. Technicians vary the energy level directed at the patient by adjusting the speed of the electrons as they hurtle toward the target.

A linear accelerator is a highly accurate and sophisticated machine that uses computers, X-ray equipment, and shielded rooms to pinpoint tumors precisely and then eliminate them. Using this type of machine, radiation therapists can treat tumors at varying depths in the body. Some tumors are near the surface—skin cancer, for example— and can be treated with lower-level energy beams. Other tumors, such as in lung cancer, are more deeply placed and so require higher levels of energy.

Table 3
Types of Radiation

Type of Radiation	Use
1. External photons and particles	
a. Low energy photons or electrons	Skin cancers, shallow lymph nodes, ribs, lip cancers, for example
b. High energy photons	Deep cancers such as lung, abdominal, or pelvic structures
2. Internal beam implants	Placed or injected into body cavities, next to a tumor
Radioactive cesium, radium, iodine, iridium, cobalt, gold, others	
3. Hyperthermia (heating body tissue)	Largely experimental, but being used together with external beam radiation therapy in large, bulky tumors
Ultrasound or sound waves; thermal or microwaves	
4. Injectable radiation	This bone-seeking radioactive drug goes to bony tumors and delivers its radiation to a specific site where it is needed. This is especially useful when prostate cancer has gone to the bone.
Strontium-89	

Are There Side Effects?

The side effects of radiation therapy usually affect only the specific area irradiated. These can include skin reactions (similar to sunburn), hair loss, and mucous membrane (such as mouth, throat, anus, and genital) irritation. Radiation can also be hard on bone marrow and blood counts. In most cases, these side effects will be temporary, but very high doses of radiation may result in permanent tissue damage. In addition, an area that has received high doses of radiation usually cannot be irradiated again because the skin "remembers" the radiation and reacts strongly against the later dose.

In the vast majority of cases, of course, the benefits of radiotherapy far outweigh the disadvantages—and recent developments have eliminated many former disadvantages. Today's radiation therapist can deliver treatment with greater accuracy and fewer side effects than ever before. In fact, radiation therapy can be so effective that it is sometimes called surgery without a knife.

Strong Medicine: The Option of Chemotherapy

But both surgery and radiation have their limitations. Each of them can remove a patch of weeds in a corner of the garden, but neither can treat the whole garden. A surgeon cannot operate throughout the body to get at all the outbreaks of a cancer as they occur, and the radiation therapist cannot irradiate the whole body to remove one tumor. Either treatment would probably kill the patient. Tumors that have spread to different parts of the body, therefore, must be treated with other methods.

Chemotherapy is used to treat cancers that have spread to more than one place in the body. The word is a shorter form of "chemical therapy." (The even shorter form used by many cancer patients and professionals is chemo.) Simply put, chemotherapy is the introduction of certain drugs or chemicals into the patient's body in an effort to eliminate cancers. (See table 4 for a list of the commonly used chemicals.)

In many types of cancer, especially those that are spread throughout the body, chemotherapy is our best means of attack. To return to the garden analogy, if cancer is the weed that has infested the whole garden, chemotherapy is the best weed killer—often the only way to cover the entire overgrown garden. Sometimes it takes just one application of a weed killer to get rid of the problem plants, and sometimes it takes many. Sometimes one kind is enough, but sometimes it takes many different kinds of chemicals.

For many people, of course, the word *chemotherapy* carries very unpleasant associations—hair loss, vomiting, weakness, and even death.

Many people think of a friend or relative who had chemotherapy while dying of cancer and assume that the chemotherapy hastened or even caused that person's death. My patients often tell me in their first visit, "I'm not going to take chemotherapy. It'll kill you!"

This kind of thinking is simply wrong. The idea that chemotherapy will kill a patient is another myth. It is true that chemotherapy has unpleasant side effects (although, as we shall see, some of these are now being minimized). But in fact, compared to dangers of allowing multiple-site cancer to grow untreated, even the most unpleasant side effects of chemotherapy are insignificant. If a patient refuses to take a round of chemotherapy that is known to be effective, he or she is allowing cancer cells to grow unchallenged and risking harm far worse than anything that chemotherapy inflicts—including death.

Instead of thinking of chemotherapy as an enemy, therefore, try to think of chemotherapy (if indicated) as a key ally in your battle against cancer. It may even help to envision the chemotherapy molecules as warriors going off to battle as they are introduced into the body. These warriors might not be perfect, and they may cause a variety of other unwanted effects, but at this point they are among our best strategies for killing the enemy.

Table 4
Drugs Used in Chemotherapy

GENERIC NAMES	TRADE NAMES
Mustards	
chlorambucil	Leukeran
cyclophosphamide	Cytoxan, Neosar
ifosfamide	IFEX/Mesnex
mechlorethamine	Mustargen, Nitrogen Mustard
melphalan	Alkeran, L-PAM
uracil mustard	Uracil Mustard
Nitrosureas	
busulfan	Myleran
carmustine	BCNU, BiCNU
lomustine	CCNU, CeeNu
streptozocin	Zanosar
Antimetabolites	
cytosine arabinoside (ARA-C)	Cytarabine, Cytosar-U, Tarabine PFS
5-fluorouracil (5-FU)	Fluorouracil, Adrucil

floxuridine	FUDR, Floxuridine
fludarabine	Fludara
gemcitabine	Gemzar
leucovorin	Wellcovorin (given with 5-fluorouracil and Methotrexate)
pentostatin	Nipent
methotrexate	Methotrexate, Folex, Rheumatrex, Mexate
6-mercaptopurine (6-MP)	Purinethol
6-thioguanine (6-TG)	Thioguanine, 6TG

Vinca Plant Products

vincristine	Oncovin, Vincasar
vinblastine	Velban
vinorelbine	Navelbine

Biologicals

erythropoietin	Epogen, Procrit
filgrastim	Neupogen
immunoglobulin	IGIV, Gammagard, Sandoglobulin
interferon	Roferon-A, IntronA, Alferon
interleukin-2	Proleukin
levamisole	Ergamisol
octreotide	Sandostatin
sargramostim	Leukine, Prokine

Podophyllotoxins

etoposide (VP-16)	Vepesid
teniposide (VM-26)	Vumon

Natural Antitumor Antibiotics

bleomycin	Blenoxane
daunorubicin	Cerubidine
doxorubicin	Adriamycin, Rubex
idarubicin	Idamycin
mithramycin	Mithracin
mitomycin	Mutamycin
mitoxantrone	Novantrone

Miscellaneous

asparaginase	Elspar
cisplatin	Platinol
carboplatin	Paraplatin
cladribine (2CDA)	Leustatin
dacarbazine	DTIC-Dome
docetaxel	Taxotere
granisetron	Kytril
hydroxyurea	Hydrea
hexamethylmelamine	Hexalen
irinotecan	Camptosar
ondansetron	Zofran
paclitaxel	Taxol
pentostatin	Nipent
procarbazine	Matulane
topotecan (CPT-11)	Hycamtin

Hormones

anastrozole	Arimidex
androgens (male hormones)	Telac, Anadrol, Nandrolone, Deca-Durabolin, Halotestin
antiestrogens (tamoxifen)	Nolvadex
corticosteroids	Prednisone, Dexamethasone, Deltasone, Medrol, Decadron
estrogens	Estrone, Estrace, DES, Estradiol, Premarin, Estraderm, Estinyl, Stilphostrol
flutamide	Eulexin
goserelin	Zoladex
leuprolide	Lupron
progestins	Megace, Megestrol, Prodox, Provera, Depo-Provera
steroid inhibitor	Cytadren, Ketoconazole, Nizoral, Mitotane
thyroid hormones	Levothyroxine, Liothyronine

Why Side Effects Happen

It may help to understand why chemotherapy brings on unpleasant side effects in the first place. They are caused primarily by the fact that chemotherapy is aimed at cells that are growing out of control. But it also attacks normal cells that are trying to grow—hair cells, blood cells, mucous membranes, cells in the lining of the mouth and digestive tract, even fingernails. It is in these growing cells, therefore, that the side effects of chemotherapy are felt.

Hair, for example, may stop growing and even fall out but will return when chemotherapy is discontinued. Sometimes a patient's fingernails will have marks that look like the rings of a tree. A semi-circular mark reflecting each round of chemotherapy may darken the normally pink fingernail.

Chemotherapy may also attack blood cells. This is why doctors closely monitor the amounts of both white and red blood cells, as well as platelets. These cells have an extraordinary variety of functions, as we saw in chapter 3. Decreased numbers of any of them (low blood counts) can lead to such difficulties as infection, weakness, abnormal bleeding tendencies, and shortness of breath.

The lining of the digestive system is also hit hard by chemotherapy. Diarrhea, mouth sores, feelings of nausea, and vomiting sometimes result.

None of these are pleasant. Sometimes they are very difficult to endure. And when you are experiencing these symptoms, it can seem as if they will never go away.

But the good news is that normal (noncancerous) tissues affected by chemotherapy can and do replenish themselves. In almost every case, hair grows back, fingernails become healthy again, blood counts are restored, and stomach lining regenerates. When a cancer cell dies, however, it is dead forever. It will never come back. If the surgery, radiation, and/or chemotherapy kills all the cancer cells, a cure will result! Although putting up with the side effects is a burdensome chore, you can see that the benefit greatly outweighs the cost.

Tables 5, 6, and 7 compare the common chemotherapy drugs in terms of their tendency to induce nausea or hair loss and their relative cost. Keep in mind, however, that the side effects of a particular drug will vary from person to person and that some drugs may have other side effects. When looking at the cost chart, keep in mind that costs vary from office to office. Don't be afraid to ask your doctor for a price list.

Table 5
Chemotherapy Drugs That May Cause Nausea

Mild	Moderate	Severe*
asparaginase	carboplatin	cisplatin
bleomycin	carmustine	dacarbazine
busulfan	cyclophosphamide	doxorubicin
chlorambucil	cytosine arabinoside	mechlorethamine
cladribine	etoposide	
5-fluorouracil	ifosfamide	
fludarabine	lomustine	
gemcitabine	mitomycin	
hydroxyurea	mitoxantrone	
interferon	procarbazine	
irinotecan	taxotere	
levamisole		
melphalan		
methotrexate		
paclitaxel		
pentostatin		
topotecan		
vinblastine		
vincristine		
vinorelbine		

*Note: The effect of all these medications can be reduced significantly when they are administered along with an antinauseant such as ondansetron (Zofran) or granesitron (Kytril).

Table 6
Chemotherapy Drugs That May Cause Hair Loss

Minimal	Moderate	Severe
bleomycin	carmustine	doxorubicin
busulfan	cyclophosphamide	etoposide
carboplatin	dacarbazine	mechlorethamine
chlorambucil	docetaxel	paclitaxel
cisplatin	ifosfamide	
5-fluorouracil	lomustine	
fludarabine	topotecan	
hydroxyurea		
interferon		
levamisole		
melphalan		
methotrexate		
mitomycin		
mitoxantrone		
procarbazine		

Table 7
Comparative Cost of Some Chemotherapy Drugs

Low	Moderate	High
5-fluorouracil	asparaginase	bleomycin
busulfan	carmustine	carboplatin
chlorambucil	cyclophosphamide	cisplatin
hydroxyurea	dacarbazine	docetaxel
lomustine	daunorubicin	doxorubicin
mechlorethamine	filgrastin	etoposide
melphalan	leucovorin	gemcitabine
methotrexate	levamisole	idarubicin
vinblastine	mitomycin	ifosfamide
vincristine	procarbazine	interferon
	sargramostin	interleukin-2
	vinorelbine	irinotecan
		mitoxantrone
		paclitaxel
		topotecan

New Strides in Chemotherapy

There is more good news. Improvements in chemotherapy are being made on two fronts to reduce the incidence of side effects. The first improvements are "smart" drugs that can reduce and sometimes eliminate the common side effect of nausea.

Nausea arises for two reasons as the result of chemotherapy. One is that the digestive tract is actually irritated by the chemotherapy. But the other is that the brain is getting a message that a horrible substance has been eaten and must be expelled. So the brain tells the digestive tract to vomit continuously until it senses that the foreign substance is gone. This can take anywhere from six hours to several days. However, some of the new smart drugs (such as ondansetron and granisetron) can turn off the brain's nausea control center even while the foreign chemical is circulating through the body. The result is that some patients receiving chemotherapy today have little problem with nausea.

A second innovation prevents patients from getting sore arms and veins. Although chemotherapy is introduced to the body through a variety of routes—including by mouth and by being injected into the skin, fat, muscle, peritoneum, pleura, or even spinal fluid—most chemotherapy is injected into veins. And this is a problem for patients with small or difficult-to-access veins or whose veins tend to pop, roll, collapse, or burst—giving fits to doctors, nurses, technicians, and patients. Doctors can now use access ports, which are really nothing more than artificial veins. They can be implanted surgically under the skin or left outside the body, taped to the skin. In either case, they are small, flexible tubes carefully inserted into larger veins in the arm or near the shoulder and used for injecting the necessary medications. They can be left in place as long as the chemotherapy is needed.

Bone-Marrow Transplants—The Atomic Bomb of Chemotherapy

If surgery, radiation, and conventional chemotherapy are not enough, physicians may turn to a newer, more radical application of chemotherapy, the bone-marrow transplant. The difference between this and traditional chemotherapy can be compared to the difference between conventional warfare and the atomic bomb. Traditional chemotherapy is like conventional warfare with ground forces, tanks, and artillery. Bone-marrow transplantation represents a quantum leap to the explosive power of an atomic warhead. It is used when other methods seem unable to stop the spread of cancer.

What does this method involve? To go back once more to our garden analogy, it is like taking a few good seeds out of the plants you want to save in your garden, then poisoning the entire garden so that everything dies—good plants and bad plants. Then, when the poison has left the garden, you go back and sow the good seeds, hoping that the bad plants (weeds) are dead forever and that the new seeds will become a healthy garden.

In much the same way, bone marrow, when it is relatively pure, can be removed and saved in a frozen state before the patient undergoes intensive chemotherapy. Once the good marrow is safely stored, the patient is subjected to extremely high doses of chemotherapy—amounts that would almost certainly be fatal without the stored marrow to replenish the blood supply. After the chemicals have been received, bone marrow is injected into the patient. Either the patient's own bone marrow can be used (an autologous transplant), or that of a closely matched donor—usually a brother or sister—can be employed (an allogeneic transplant). Much like seeds in the wind, these saved marrow cells find the perfect spot to grow and multiply, replenishing the patient's depleted blood with healthy blood produced by new, growing bone marrow.

This sounds like a very risky procedure, and it is, but not nearly as risky as it used to be. Thousands are done every year with positive results. Bone-marrow transplantation has been used to treat acute and chronic leukemias, lymphomas, and Hodgkin's disease. It is also being tried for a variety of solid tumors such as ovary, testicle, breast, and lung cancers. As a general rule, this procedure is performed after other treatments have failed or when the tumor has a very high likelihood of returning after remission.

Because of its very high cost, insurance companies may limit their coverage. For instance, they tend to cover this treatment only for cancers that have better chances of recovery. That is, they may cover bone marrow transplants for chronic myelogenous leukemia, but not for metastatic ovarian cancer. We suggest that you ask your doctor or insurance representative if bone-marrow transplant is available to you as a covered benefit.

Going "Natural": The Option of Biological Therapy

The fourth major type of cancer therapy is very new. Only recently has it left the laboratory and been used on patients. Its idea is to use substances that our body normally makes to fight cancer. More specifically, in this type of therapy, scientists use the genes from our chromosomes (see chapter 1) to create proteins that the body normally makes to kill unwanted cells. These proteins are then targeted specifically to attack cancer cells.

To get an idea of how this works, we need to switch the garden analogy around a little and talk about pest control instead of weed control. An organic gardener, for instance, would not use a pesticide to rid the garden of Japanese beetles but a pheromone or sex-attractant to lure the insects into a plastic bag where they can be trapped and killed. Similarly, the biologicals use the body's natural way of fighting unwanted cells to try to kill cancer cells.

Before we describe some of these forms of biological therapy, we must stress that many of them are still in early stages of development and are either unavailable to cancer patients or must be received at a university hospital. They have varying and unpredictable response rates. Some are quite toxic, and others are simply too new to understand and use. We trust, however, that in years to come these methods will become both more predictable and more widely available.

Monoclonal Antibodies

One of the first and the best-known biological therapies is the use of monoclonal antibodies. An antibody is a protein manufactured by the white blood cells that attacks an unwanted substance in the body—a cell, a virus, or another antibody. A monoclonal antibody is a clone (copy) of a single antibody made in large numbers.

Scientists have discovered how to create monoclonal antibodies through genetic engineering and to put them to use in very accurate and specific ways. The antibodies are manufactured with the ability to find their targets, attack them, and generally ignore surrounding tissues. The intent is to attach a lethal poison to monoclonal antibodies, and then inject them into the body. The antibodies would attach themselves to their specific target, a cancer cell, and then release their baggage (the poison) into the target to do its work.

Unfortunately, this process has generally not worked very well up to this point. The idea is good, but it must be made to adapt to the body's immune system, which is enormously complex. So far, researchers have not been able to make the necessary adaptations. But they are still working, and a breakthrough may be around the corner. So keep watching the newspaper for reports on monoclonal antibody research.

Gene Therapy

A second biological therapy that may be in the news for the next few years is gene therapy. You may recall that in chapter 1 we said that it is usually the gene, or the basic information unit of the chromosome, that goes haywire in a cancer cell. It follows that if a gene (in this case, an oncogene) is completely understood, then a doctor should be able to fix it. Just as a mechanic can replace or repair a defective part in an otherwise sound engine, a gene therapist should be able to go into a cell to fix a bad gene so that the cell can revert to its normal state.

There are already many diseases, both malignant and nonmalignant, in which the defective gene is known. These include hemophilia A, diabetes, certain forms of dwarfism, and a rare childhood eye tumor called retinoblastoma. But this doesn't mean you can run out and ask your doctor for a gene replacement! Isolating the defective gene is just the first step in being able to fix it. Even though we know which gene causes diabetes, for instance, we are still a long way from knowing how to repair the gene.

In the 1990s, gene therapy is just in its beginning stages and has been applied successfully only in some noncancerous childhood diseases (such as Severe Combined Immunodeficiency Syndrome, or SCIDS). It may be years before gene therapy is added to our list of commonly used biological treatments for cancer. Nevertheless, I (Bill) expect it will be used on some of my patients before I close my career as an oncologist.

Other Biological Agents

Other forms of biological therapy include interferons, interleukins, tumor vaccines, colony-stimulating factors, T-lymphocytes, and tumor necrosis factors. Like the therapies we have already discussed, these are natural body cells or proteins that have been manipulated by scientists to be used to the patient's advantage.

Interferons are proteins, manufactured naturally by the body's cells, that activate the immune system when an enemy is perceived. They can be manufactured through gene technology and used to treat certain rare conditions such as hairy cell leukemia, chronic myelogenous leukemia, and Kaposi's sarcoma (a cancer of the connective tissue associated with AIDS).

Colony-stimulating factors (CSF) are hormones that instruct the bone marrow to make red or white blood cells. These can be used to help prevent infections resulting from low blood counts after chemotherapy. They are administered by injection to strengthen the bone marrow's ability to make white blood cells and thus shorten the period of time that patients risk infection after chemotherapy. One of our great hopes is that they may make it possible to give larger doses of chemotherapy over shorter periods of time and therefore cure more cancers.

The other biological agents listed above are now being tried in experimental cancer centers and are not available for routine use.

One day these biological therapies may be the silver bullet that all of us who treat cancer dream of. That is, they may be able to seek out a cancer cell, kill it, and leave the surrounding tissues alone. But until that silver bullet is perfected, we must rely on the other proven therapies. Though not universally effective, they have saved thousands of lives, and we can be thankful for them.

Working with Your Doctor

Because of the wide range of cancer treatments available, you and your doctor have some important decisions to make. As you work together to make these decisions and carry out the treatment, it may be very helpful to understand the full range of opinions.

A Range of Opinions—But One Anchor

Many hospitals use what is called a tumor board (or tumor conference) to facilitate this discussion process. This is a panel of many different kinds of medical specialists who meet to discuss each case. At their meetings, the pathology slides, X rays, and other details of the case are presented and discussed openly. The gathering of learned opinions from all the relevant specialties is your optimal bet for determining the best treatment for your cancer.

You may also be asked to see a variety of physicians—a surgeon, a radiation oncologist, a medical oncologist, or others—before starting your therapy. This is not to help the physicians involved make more money. It is simply the wisest way to get the best range of perspectives for your specific case.

But while it is important to seek out a full range of opinions, it is equally as important to have one doctor who will serve as your anchor and coordinator. Otherwise you may head off in many directions because of differing suggestions and be left hopelessly confused. You need one doctor to take responsibility for your case and keep the big picture in mind. This doctor will sort out all the advice you have been given and help you decide what course to follow.

Thus it is important to choose the right doctor. You should choose someone who seems trustworthy, communicates well, and thoroughly understands your particular kind of cancer. He or she must be willing to spend appropriate time with you to answer your questions. (A good doctor will never be bothered if you take notes or write questions down.)

What to Ask

You should feel free to ask your oncologist any questions that occur to you, including the following:

- Can this cancer be put into remission? (Remission is defined as the state when there are no apparent traces of the cancer remaining.)

- How long can remission last? Is it possible for me to be cured?

- Do I need surgery? Is it necessary to remove the diseased organ, or can a partial removal accomplish the same result? (Often this is done in conjunction with radiation.)

- Will I need chemotherapy? If so, will I receive one chemotherapy drug or several in combination?

- How many months of chemotherapy does my kind of cancer typically require?

- Will the drugs be given orally, intravenously, or by some other route?

- Can the chemotherapy itself cause cancer at a later date?

- Will I need radiation therapy?

- What side effects can I expect from my surgery, my medication, or my radiation? What can I do to cope with these side effects?

- Will I become sterile as a result of my treatment? Are there ways to preserve my fertility?

- How quickly will I know if the treatment is working? What tests will be done to measure a response?

- Will my blood count fall as a result of my treatment? Do I have to worry about infections?

- Is there a possibility that I will require blood transfusions during my chemotherapy?

- What is the risk of getting infected or diseased blood from a transfusion?

- Can I refuse surgery and still be your patient?

- Do I have the right to stop radiation anytime I want?

- Do I have the right to stop chemotherapy if I choose?

- Are there any new therapies, such as natural therapies, available to me and appropriate to my illness? How can I gain access to these?*

---

*Feel free to photocopy this list of questions and take it with you on your next visit to the doctor.

In this one short chapter, we have explored the entire range of cancer therapies. We make no pretense, however, of providing exhaustive treatment options; entire books have been written on the tiniest fragments of this topic. We hope we have given you a basic understanding of how these four treatments differ from one another, how they work on cancer cells, and how they will affect you. If we have completely ruined your desire to ever garden again, we offer our humble apologies!

6

What Are My Rights?

What to Expect As a Cancer Patient

What do you as a cancer patient (or the loved one of a cancer patient) have a right to expect from your doctors, nurses, and therapists? And what do those caregivers have a right to expect from you?

Before we talk specifics, perhaps we should discuss just what we mean by rights. Rights can be understood in two ways—legal and moral. A legal right is a claim upheld by law. If Joe agrees to pay Tom a hundred dollars to fix his car and then fails to pay after Tom has made the repairs, the law will support Tom's efforts to get Joe to keep his side of the agreement. The law, in other words, says that Tom has a right to the one hundred dollars.

It is widely believed that there are moral rights as well as legal rights. That is, there are claims a person has a right to make, regardless of whether that person's society has enshrined those claims in a law.

The American Declaration of Independence, for instance, pronounces that every human being has a right to life, liberty, and the pursuit of happiness. The thirteen American colonies in the eighteenth century declared that they had a right to certain liberties, such as representation, despite laws that the British government had passed in an effort to curtail those liberties.

We believe that the cancer patient has both a legal and moral right to good medical care. The patient has a legal right because he or she has presumably paid—either through insurance, cash, or barter—for the doctor's services. That financial agreement, protected by law, implicitly stipulates that in return for payment the doctor will provide the best care possible.

But even if there were no legal right, the cancer patient would have a moral right to good medical care. That is, even if the patient is poor and without insurance, he has a right to good treatment. Because a doctor's profession is dedicated to healing the sick, and because the cancer patient is a human being in legitimate need, justice and decency require that the doctor give the patient the best possible care. This is an appeal not to benevolence and charity from the doctor but to universal human standards of justice and equality. These are standards below which a human should not be allowed to fall.

We believe, therefore, that when you agree with your doctor to receive care for your cancer, you have a variety of rights as a patient. These include:

Right #1: The Best Care Possible

You have a right to the best care your community can offer. This might seem obvious, but there is more to this statement than you might think. It does not say that you have a right to expect the best health care on earth, nor does it say that your doctor must be the smartest or the best educated doctor in town. But it does say that you can insist on the best care possible in your city, even if it means that your doctor must consult with other specialists. Many times it is more important to keep an average doctor who is a good communicator and friend than to seek out a better-known physician who does not know you, your family, or your history. If your average doctor is a strong advocate for your medical interests, if he or she communicates well and knows when to seek assistance, then that doctor can most likely deliver to you the best care available in your community.

Right #2: Clear Explanations

After you have described all of your ailments and the doctor has examined you, you have a right to receive good and thorough explanations of (1) the doctor's initial diagnosis, (2) the recommended tests, (3) the suggested therapy, and (4) your prognosis (expected outcome of the treatment).

Exactly What Is Wrong with Me?

Imagine that your doctor—with whom you have spoken for a total of five minutes—enters your room and announces, "You have a pheochromocytoma that needs surgical extirpation." Believe it or not, there are some patients who would simply reply, "Oh," and hope the doctor would do the right thing. The wise patient, however, will demand a full explanation of these mysterious words. Your diagnosis is the key to everything else that happens to you—the testing, the treatment, and the outcome. You have a right to an explanation in understandable language of just what the doctor thinks is wrong with you.

Why Are You Ordering This Test?

You have a right to understand why you are having a certain test and what that test entails. Lawyers have a name for the situation in which a doctor orders a painful test without explanation or the patient's permission; they call it assault and battery! Now very few doctors have actually been indicted for assault and battery, but the term rightfully suggests that a test can be invasive, potentially painful, and possibly dangerous. The patient, therefore, has the right to understand ahead of time what the test will involve—and the right to refuse it.

The task of explaining a test is often delegated to a nurse or a physician's assistant. If that suits you, fine. But if you would like a full explanation from your personal physician, don't hesitate to ask for it. You have a right to an explanation before you must endure any test.

Exactly What Will Happen to Me?

You have a right to understand your proposed treatment, including its potential side effects. In fact, you should be able to get printed literature from your doctor explaining the treatment and possible side effects.

We must warn, however, that knowing all the potential side effects is not always possible and sometimes may not even be advisable. I (Bill) know a doctor who prescribed the common drug prednisone. Before giving it to the patient, he explained most of its common side effects, such as elevated blood sugars, elevated blood pressure, and the development of cataracts, acne, and obesity. But he failed to mention one of the many rare side effects: aggravation of hip arthritis. As it turned out, the patient wound up needing hip replacement surgery.

Was the doctor negligent in not explaining every remote side effect? It is doubtful that he could have explained all of them in any sort of coherent manner. It is also questionable whether every patient should know every potential side effect, particularly those that are not likely to arise. To do so would simply alarm the patient unnecessarily.

Because we live in a society that has seen marvelous medical advances and enjoys immediate gratification of most of our needs, we tend to expect perfection from our doctors and hospitals. But should we? Should we be surprised that our health care will sometimes be painful? That there will sometimes be unforeseen side effects?

Our point is that you have a right to understand your treatment and its side effects, but you do not have a right to expect perfect treatment devoid of side effects. We live in an imperfect world. Any treatment you receive may fail, and may even harm you, but that is never the expectation of the doctor ordering it. The doctor expects that the treatment will make you better, with a tolerable set of side effects. Your right is to be satisfied with an understanding of the treatment and a reasonable range of possible side effects.

What Are My Chances?

You have a right to your doctor's best estimate of your chances of remission. We use the word *remission* here because it is often more meaningful than cure. In fact, I tell my patients that the word *remission* is the prettiest word in the English language. Remission means there is no evidence of remaining cancer after the end of treatment. For most cancers, the doctor can give you very accurate estimates of the chances of achieving remission.

Cure, on the other hand, implies that the cancer is completely gone and that your doctor knows what the future will bring. But no doctor has a crystal ball that can assure you absolutely that the cancer will never return, any more than your mechanic can guarantee what your car will do in the month following a repair. While remission is the goal of many cancer therapies, cure is up to God.

You have a right, in other words, to your doctor's best estimate of your chances for remission. But you do not have a right to having those predictions come true. Your doctor is human, and M.D. does not stand for "Minor Diety"!

Right #3: To Stop If You Want To

You always have a right to discontinue a test or treatment at any time. A test or treatment may turn out to be different from what was explained. Since you are the sole owner of your body, you alone should decide whether to continue with the treatment. Even if your doctor insists that stopping would be against his or her wishes, you have every right to make that decision.

Right #4: A Second Opinion

You have a right to see another doctor to get a second opinion. This seems obvious to many people, but others feel that seeking advice from another doctor would somehow be a breach of ethics. This is not the case. A good doctor will not be embarrassed or threatened if a patient seeks another opinion. In fact, as a practicing physician, I feel that a second opinion helps me in two ways. If the other doctor agrees with me, that agreement simply confirms my original thinking. If the doctor disagrees with me, his disagreement shows me I may be wrong. I then consider this an opportunity to reexamine my own diagnosis and perhaps to learn from the other doctor.

Many times, of course, a disagreement is a matter not of right and wrong, but of differences in philosophy. Consider a treatment for disease X, for which six months of therapy is known to help only one out of ten patients. One doctor may feel that it is not worth subjecting nine people to the therapy for the sake of just one. Another doctor may feel that helping one is a worthy goal and so will treat all ten, since the physician does not know which one of the ten will be helped.

If a doctor tells you not to get a second opinion or seems threatened by your request, that is reason in itself to get one. You owe it to yourself to make sure your doctor's advice is sound. If for any reason you are not satisfied with the care you are receiving—physically, emotionally, or even spiritually—you should at least explore the option of a second opinion.

Right #5: Access to Your Records

You have a right to view—and obtain copies of—any of your medical records. This includes X rays and all other tests that have been performed. Your medical record is exactly that—your medical record. There may be a charge for copying, but the information that has been collected about your body, in print or on film, should never be hidden from you.

Right #6: Ongoing Care

In the event that cancer therapies have failed or been discontinued, you have a right to not be abandoned by your physician. If your physician feels more treatment would not help you, he or she may choose to refer you to another physician. But it is not your doctor's prerogative to prevent you from seeing him or her for morphine, further treatment, or simply a brief chat if you so desire. You can expect, and should get, quality care after cancer therapies have stopped.

Right #7: A Little Respect

You have a right to be treated with dignity. There are times when health care professionals forget their patients' need for respect. In such times, they need to be reminded that a patient should never be laughed at, belittled, ignored, or ridiculed. They need to remember that there are few things as elevating as being listened to and cared for and few things so degrading as being ignored or ridiculed. If a doctor or nurse or other health-care professional tramples on your personal dignity, don't be afraid to speak up.

One little way in which many American hospitals attack their patients' self-respect is to require them to wear oversized napkins (patient gowns) that expose their private parts for all the world to see. There is no reason why you cannot insist on wearing your own pajamas when you have to stay in the hospital. They help you retain your dignity and identity while at the same time bringing a bit of warmth from home into a sterile hospital room.

Right #8: Something for the Pain

You have a right to have something done to relieve pain. Not all the hurts that go with cancer and its treatment can be relieved, but you have a right to ask your doctor to at least try.

There is a difference, however, between pain and suffering. Pain can often be relieved with narcotics, but suffering is a feeling deep inside that narcotics cannot touch. I tell my patients that I can try to relieve their pain, but that I don't have a pill for their suffering. The deep hurt that comes when a patient realizes that treatment has been unsuccessful is something that no physician can relieve.

It is at this point that some patients or their loved ones think of suicide. And it is for these people, particularly, that chapter 14 was written. For we are convinced that suffering—even the suffering that comes from cancer—has meaning, and that patients who can find that meaning can also find the strength to endure. We hope and pray that those who read this book, especially chapters 9 through 12, will find help for their suffering.

Suicide is not the answer. You may have a number of rights as a cancer patient, but you do not have the right to determine when death will occur—even for yourself. These are not decisions that doctors can make either; at times it is even dangerous to speculate about them. That decision is a matter for God alone.

Your doctor has a duty to inform you of your chances of remission, but those chances are based only on the statistics of hundreds or thousands of patients who have had a similar cancer before you. Your cancer is unique. Although others have had the same kind of cancer, that cancer has never before occurred in this particular patient: you. So, in a sense, your cancer will write a new history in you. Your doctor, then, has a duty to give you a best guess of your chances, but it is only a guess. And doctors' guesses in these matters are often wrong.

More Rights—And Some Responsibilities

The cancer patient's rights doubtless extend far beyond what we have sketched in this chapter. Some cancer survivors, for example, have encountered discrimination in the workplace because of their experience with cancer. For information about your legal rights concerning employment, you may want to contact your local chapter of the American Cancer Society.

Even as you are becoming informed of your rights, however, it is important to remember that your doctor has rights as well. He or she has a right to expect you to show up for appointments, to take your medicines as directed (if possible), to keep a positive outlook, and to do what you can to stay strong—eat right, get enough exercise and sleep, avoid undue stress, and so on.

Too often a patient expects a cure from simply swallowing a tablet or getting an injection. But it takes cooperation from both sides to maximize chances for full recovery.

7

How Do I Pay My Bills?

Insurance, Medicare, and Other Strategies

The greatest fear many cancer patients face is not debilitation or even death, but the inability to pay their bills.

Some may have prided themselves on their financial management, but now something has arisen that may ruin their reputation and ruin them financially. Worse yet, they fear that they are saddling their families with debt. (Their families are probably frightened as well.)

Other patients and families are simply overwhelmed with confusion as the bills and EOBs (explanations of benefits) mount ever higher. It all seems complicated, so difficult to understand. And it hits at a time when they are also trying to cope with frightening diagnoses, strange-sounding treatments, and uncomfortable side effects.

The purpose of this chapter is to dispel some of the fear and confusion that accompany the financial aspects of cancer. It may introduce you to some sources of funding you didn't know existed. It should show that most cancer patients in the United States who have health insurance can afford cancer care—and that there is even hope for those who do not have insurance.

The High Cost of Health Care

The crux of the problem for most of us is the enormous cost of health care in America. One reason for this is our demand for the best. We want the best health care available, and, fortunately, many of us can get it. In general, American health care is the most technologically advanced health care in the world. But the price for getting the best care is very high, and it goes up every year.

In 1954, the per capita expenditure for health care in this country was $176. By 1988, that figure had increased to $2,124—an elevenfold increase. During that thirty-four-year period, health care expenditures grew from 5.9 percent of the gross national product to 11.1 percent.

There is no foreseeable end to such increases. As long as researchers continue to develop new technology to keep us alive longer and longer, the costs will keep rising higher and higher.

With costs increasing each year, more people find themselves unable to pay for medical services. In this chapter we will look at the most common strategies such people use to get their medical bills paid. Then we'll try to help you make some sense of the paperwork involved and warn you of problems that may arise. Finally, we'll discuss the problem of people who have no insurance.

Strategies to Pay the Bills

It is not unusual today for a visit to the doctor to cost several hundred dollars and for a prescription to cost well over a hundred. With costs like these for such simple services, it is apparent that most Americans cannot afford to use the traditional fee-for-service method of payment. We can usually pay the mechanic after a car repair, but it is increasingly impossible for most of us, relying entirely on our own resources, to pay the doctor and hospital for the enormously expensive treatment we need for cancer. This is why many Americans are thankful for such resources as private health insurance, government insurance such as Medicare and Medicaid, or managed health care systems such as HMOs.

Private Health Insurance

The concept behind private health insurance is that if enough people pay monthly premiums into a pool, when someone gets sick, there is enough money to pay for treatment. What this means, in effect, is that those who never get sick pay the bills of those who do. This arrangement might be somewhat inequitable, but most people are happy to participate for the peace of mind that comes with knowing that if they face catastrophic illness, at least the majority of their bills will be paid.

There are many different kinds of private health insurance. Their costs and benefits vary greatly, depending on factors such as the participants' age, health, and risk of illness to come. Large insurance companies, such as Blue Cross/Blue Shield, often offer widely different plans to appeal to different needs and differing abilities to pay premiums.

Many insurance plans are offered through companies or other large groups that are able to pool resources and obtain better terms.

Most plans do not pay for everything. Many medical services are covered at an 80 percent rate after a deductible. That is, after a patient has paid the first, say, $150 a year for medical treatment, the insurance company pays 80 percent of the remaining fees. The patient pays the remaining 20 percent, which is called the patient's copayment.

Sometimes there is a cap on out-of-pocket expenses (the money that comes out of the pocket of the insured patient), so patients know they will not have to pay more than a maximum amount for a given year or a given illness. On the other hand, there is sometimes a lifetime maximum (the total amount that will be paid, regardless of actual expense) for certain diseases. And some services are not covered at all. Mammograms, for instance, are noncovered (an out-of-pocket expense) in many insurance plans.

Many cancer prevention tests, such as mammograms and Pap

smears, are now mandated for annual insurance coverage in some states. For information about such regulations in your area, you may want to check with your local chapter of the American Cancer Society or your state insurance regulatory board.

Government Health Insurance

Because of rapidly escalating health costs, private insurance is becoming more and more expensive. In fact, it is growing beyond the reach of many who are self-employed. Even people who work for others are often uninsured or underinsured because their employers are unable or unwilling to provide complete coverage. For a limited number of these people, the two forms of government-provided health insurance—Medicare and Medicaid—provide a desperately needed safety net.

Medicare: Part A

Medicare is a way of paying hospital and doctor bills for United States citizens who are either disabled or above sixty-five years of age. It also provides coverage for those who need permanent kidney dialysis.

Part A of Medicare insurance pays for inpatient hospital care, a limited number of outpatient services, care at skilled nursing homes, home health care, and approved hospice care. Services covered include use of a semiprivate room (it will not pay for a private room unless your doctor deems it medically necessary), meals, nursing care, intensive care when necessary, pharmaceuticals (medicine), and blood transfusions.

What is not covered by Medicare?

- Custodial care or those activities of daily living that most people can help with, like changing linens, getting dressed, cooking meals, or even getting to the bathroom

- Nonskilled nursing home services

- Routine medical checkups, except Pap smears and mammograms

- Prescription drugs

- Service outside the United States

Medicare provides help through one of two methods: the traditional fee-for-service system or a new plan called managed care (discussed later in this chapter).

Most people do not pay any premium for Part A, but there are deductibles to be met and copayments to be made, especially if the traditional fee-for-service method of payment is chosen. These are explained in the Medicare Handbook, issued by the government, which you can obtain through your local hospital, local business administration, local social security administration office, or by calling the social security toll-free number: 1-800-772-1213.

In the early 1980s, the federal government started a new system of payment called the prospective payment system (PPS). Under this arrangement, the government pays hospitals based on a predetermined average number of days (based on regional averages) for treating people with a particular diagnosis. Take breast cancer, for example. If the prescribed treatment is a mastectomy, and if mastectomy patients in your region of the country average a 3.5-day stay in the hospital, the government will pay the hospital for 3.5 days of work whether the patient actually stay 2 days, 3.5 days, or 15 days. Because there is no way for the hospital to recover its losses after a long stay, many hospital administrators try to monitor lengths of stay under this prospective payment system because not doing so could mean huge losses for the hospital.

Medicare: Part B

Part B of Medicare pays for doctors' services, some outpatient hospital services, X-ray and laboratory tests, and medical devices such as wheelchairs and hospital beds. It does not pay for routine physical examinations, foot and dental care, prescription eyeglasses, or most immunizations.

Unlike Part A, which is paid for through our FICA payroll taxes,

Part B is not government subsidized and requires a monthly premium. Like Part A, it has an annual deductible and copayments if the traditional method of payment is chosen. If the managed care or HMO style of Medicare is chosen, insureds will continue to pay a Part B monthly premium; however, copayments are less and out-of-pocket expenses are usually less. U.S. citizens over age sixty-five can pay premiums to receive the benefits of Part B even if they don't participate in Part A. If, for example, they have private insurance to cover hospitalization, they can still use Part B to pay for doctors' fees.

Part B of Medicare pays only 80 percent of the approved (by the Medicare system) charge for the service you receive. For a cancer examination, for instance, a doctor may charge $100. But Medicare may have already decided that $60 is the approved charge for this service. That means that the government will pay 80 percent of the $60 ($48) and the covered patient must pay the other 20 percent, or $12. For that reason, most people choose to pay for additional insurance, often called Medigap insurance, which helps them meet deductibles and copayments. Medigap insurance plans vary but often cover a broad range of services typically not covered by Medicare, including prescription drugs, eyeglasses, and some screening tests.

A doctor who accepts Medicare assignment agrees by signature on a Medicare form to accept the approved charge as the total charge for that service. If your doctor normally charges $100 for a service and he or she is paid only $60, the doctor has implicitly agreed to write off the difference of $40. Of course, your doctor also expects you to pay $12 (your 20 percent of the $60), either by supplemental private insurance (such as that offered by the American Association of Retired People or Blue Cross/Blue Shield) or from your own pocket.

If your doctor has not agreed to accept Medicare assignment, then he or she expects you to pay not only the $12, but some of the additional $40 as well. That is, the doctor does not accept Medicare's estimation that $60 is a reasonable fee for the service, and he or she expects to be paid more than $60. That means you must pay the difference, either through supplemental insurance or from out-of-pocket cash. (If you are not confused by now, either you are a genius, or you have been subjected to this painful process.)

Now you can see why it is a good idea to get a list of the Medicare-participating physicians in your area. Because physicians are not required to participate in most states, there is considerable variation among doctors. Some accept Medicare assignment; many don't.

You should know, too, that the rules for Medicare change from year to year. What was true in 1995 may not be true in 1999 or 2000. There are also considerable differences from region to region. What may be true for a city may not be true for a rural area. Check your Medicare Handbook for particulars (but be sure your handbook is up to date). If you have a problem with receiving your benefits, talk to the local Medicare office. If that does not help, contact your local congressman or senator.

Medicaid

Although the names Medicare and Medicaid are similar and both are governmental health insurance programs, the similarities stop there. The purpose of Medicaid is to help the poorest of the poor. Payment for services is usually lower than any other health insurance plan. For this reason, many doctors and hospitals are less than eager to see Medicaid patients walk through their doors.

Many other doctors, however, feel a civic and moral duty to serve Medicaid patients, as well as patients who have no insurance. So for doctors who already care for more than their fair share of patients with no insurance and little or no money, a Medicaid patient can be a welcome sight. If you qualify for Medicaid and want to receive its benefits, you will want to find a list of doctors in your area who participate in the program. (Look in your phone book under state government Information Services or Medical Assistance Services.)

Medicaid programs vary from state to state because, although both federal and state tax dollars support the programs, they are administered by state governments. Each state has its own guidelines. The 1997 Virginia Medicaid Plan, for example, offers its services to seventeen different categories of people who qualify to receive full Medicaid benefits, and other categories of people who qualify for partial benefits. Even with all those categories, however, there are many people who struggle financially but whose income is too high to qualify. If you need Medicaid assistance and think you may qualify, contact your local Department of Social Services.

Once you are covered under the Medicaid program, you will need to check whether your doctor and local hospital participate. You will also need to see exactly what is covered by your state. Some states, for example, cover some prescription drugs, while others don't cover any. (Call the Medicaid office, which is usually listed with other state government phone numbers, for a Medicaid Handbook.)

Managed Health Care

The term managed health care applies to a variety of plans that offer alternatives to traditional health insurance. The two most important are Health Maintenance Organizations (HMOs) and Preferred Provider Organizations (PPOs). Both plans were created in order to save money by combining preventive health care and more efficient use of health resources. They grew out of the desire to control spiraling medical costs and have proliferated rapidly since the failure of efforts to expand government-subsidized medicine. Once offered only in larger cities, managed care plans are now available in small cities as well and are even being suggested as models to help Medicare and Medicaid control their costs.

Managed care organizations operate on a membership basis and usually offer their members treatment from a limited pool of health-care professionals. Some managed health care systems require their members to pay only a membership premium, so there are no bills or fees for services. Others charge, in addition to a membership premium, small copayments and per-visit deductibles. Most of these fees are considerably smaller than comparable payments charged by the traditional fee-for-service system. Many HMO and PPO plans offer an expanded range of services, particularly those aimed at disease prevention, in the belief that "an ounce of prevention is worth a pound of cure." Many, even those subsidized by the government, also provide for prescription drugs, screening visits, and eyeglasses. Almost all plans list the medical services they do not cover.

Another unique feature of these organizations is that they offer built-in incentives for the organization to save money through a combination of efficient practices and illness prevention. Patient premiums are paid either by an individual or an employer and make up most of the organizations' income. The fewer times doctors are consulted, X-rays are taken, and laboratory tests are conducted, therefore, the more money the plan's treasury will have at the end of the year. Whereas the standard fee-for-service system is more profitable when patients are seen often, managed health-care programs are more profitable when patients are seen less often. Hence, when HMO members stay well, the plan does well.

To cut costs, these organizations often use lower-paid paraprofessionals—nurse practitioners, physician's assistants, and registered nurses—to care for less serious cases. They also tend to limit the use of expensive technology. Rather than encouraging the use of enormously costly machinery, they are more careful to ensure that it is used only when necessary.

As you can see, these organizations have advantages and disadvantages. They help prevent wasteful use of health care by rewarding providers according to appropriate use rather than simple volume. In many instances they also promote preventive medicine and early intervention because the lower prices encourage people to seek help at the first sign that something is wrong. There is a danger, however, that in an effort to prevent loss of profit, these organizations may refrain from using some personnel or procedures that could provide genuine help.

The benefit to you of participating in a managed health-care organization is that, once you are a member, you will have less worry about new bills that you cannot pay. What you need to watch out for, though, is that your doctor and your insurance organization agree on what care is necessary. And you need to be aware that your choice of health-care providers and hospitals may be limited to those approved by the organization. When you choose between traditional fee-for-service medicine and managed care plans, you are deciding which is more important: the freedom of choice offered by fee-for-service plans, or the cost savings (and more restricted access to health care) of HMO and PPO plans. Read carefully before you sign on the dotted line.

A final word of caution. Managed health-care organizations vary widely in their approach to finances. Many involve little out-of-pocket expense, while others offer economy plans whose membership premiums are quite low but whose copayments may be high. Be sure you know all the restrictions before you join one of these organizations.

Understanding the Bills

Once you understand something about insurance, your next task will be to make sense of the blizzard of paper that starts coming in the mail once you've become involved with cancer treatment. (By the way, there is typically much less paperwork in managed care plans). In the traditional fee-for-services plans, the health provider will expect to be paid. Ignoring these growing piles of paper may seem tempting, but it is in your best interest to resist that temptation. If insurance payments are late or don't come at all, your doctor and hospital will come to you, expecting you to resolve the problem.

If you discover that the insurance company will indeed pay but later than your doctor or hospital expects, go to your doctor and hospital and explain the situation. Ask them if they can wait. Many times they can and will appreciate your effort to explain. If they won't wait, you may be forced to write them a check and be reimbursed later by your insurance company.

The mail you receive usually comes in two forms:

1. EOBs from your insurance company

2. Bills (or statements) from your doctor and hospital

EOBs (explanations of benefits) are sent from your insurance company to tell you that the doctor or hospital has filed a claim for services performed. They typically tell you the dates of services and who performed them, and they should also tell you whether the services are covered by your insurance.

Bills (or statements) tell you how much you owe; sometimes they also tell you what you (or your insurance company) have paid so far. If you are having problems paying on time, they may also show how close your account may be to being sent to a collection agency.

Try to develop a simple but workable system for filing these notices as they come and keeping track of what you owe and what you have paid. It may help to staple the EOB to the bill, so that for each service you have both the insurance form and the doctor's invoice. When you make a payment, note the date and the amount on your copy of the invoice. If you don't get a copy to keep and a copy to send with payment, take the time to get the payment photocopied as a record.

Avoiding—and Solving—Problems with Your Bills

Because the process of paying your cancer treatment bills involves so much paperwork and so many interactions between doctor, hospital, insurance company, and patient, many problems can arise. Perhaps the best way to handle these difficulties is to be alert to what forms they might take. Then you can be on guard against them and either prevent them before they arise, or at least be better prepared to face them. What follows, then, is a description of the most common problems that arise for cancer patients trying to pay their bills.

Services Not Covered

You may find that certain services provided by your doctor may not be covered in the fine print of your insurance plan. This means that you may have to pay for these services out of your own pocket. To avoid this, be sure to check ahead of time to see if your insurance covers a particular test or treatment. If it doesn't, ask your doctor if the procedure is absolutely necessary.

More Than Your Policy Will Pay

The service fee charged by your doctor or hospital may be more than the specified amount allowed by your insurance plan, thus requiring a larger copayment from you. This is particularly likely if you are a Medicare or Medicaid patient. If your doctor and hospital accept assignment for Medicare and/or Medicaid patients, then there is no problem. If not, you will need to pay the difference or work out some other arrangement.

Disputes Between Insurance Companies

If you have more than one insurance plan, each of which would normally cover the same bill, the companies may argue among themselves over which should pay, delaying payment. It may help to call your primary insurance provider and insist that the dispute be settled so the bills will be paid in a timely fashion.

What about My Cancer Policy?

Some patients have a separate cancer policy in addition to their regular health plan. A cancer policy will usually send money directly to you; it is then your responsibility to pay your doctor and hospital bills. Cancer policies are usually used as supplements to traditional insurance, as a way to help pay out-of-pocket expenses or make up for lost income.

Preauthorization Problems

Sometimes your insurance company may deny payment because you did not fulfill preauthorization requirements. Some plans have fine print requiring you to get authorization from the company before you receive a particular service. If you don't, they will not pay for the service. Before undergoing a procedure, check your policy for such a requirement and be sure to get preauthorization if it is required.

Technical Delays

Your insurance company may delay payment because of technical problems with your documentation. Sometimes, in fact, it may seem they are picking through your paperwork with a fine-tooth comb, looking for problems. This may delay payment for three, six, or even nine months after treatment. In the meantime, the bills from your doctor and hospital may be getting nastier in tone.

Some doctors and hospitals turn bills over to collection agencies after three months. If that happens to you, you may get a black mark on your credit record. To prevent this from occurring, make a point of staying in communication with your doctor and hospital. Ask them to talk to you before they send any bill to a collection agency. Tell them that you are trying to arrange payment, and ask them for more time if it is needed. If worse comes to worst, you may have to write a check to pay the bill and wait to get reimbursed later. (Many doctors and hospitals accept major credit cards.)

Case Managers

You may get a call or letter from a nurse or doctor, not connected with your treatment, who says he or she is a case manager. This is a person, often a registered nurse, hired by your insurance company for the purpose of cutting costs. The case manager is not a member of your medical team but may intervene in your treatment to make sure the insurance company is not being overcharged. In most cases, a case manager will not present a problem, and he or she may indeed prevent unnecessary costs to you and your insurance company. Sometimes, however, a case manager will try to get your doctor and hospital to cut corners and not give you the treatment your doctor thinks you need. In that case, encourage your doctor to insist on the best treatment.

Unapproved or Experimental Drugs

You may receive a notice from your insurance company that a certain drug is unapproved or experimental. Don't be alarmed until you have checked this out. Most likely, you are not getting dangerous or ineffective therapy from your doctor. Instead, one of several things is probably happening:

- Your insurance company may not be abreast of the latest drug research. It may not have heard of your doctor's therapy because it has only recently been shown to be effective.

- Your doctor may be using the drug in an off label manner. The Food and Drug Administration (FDA), a branch of the United States government, reviews drugs for safety and effectiveness before releasing them on the market. The drugs are then labeled as approved. It is common for doctors to use drugs in innovative (and often more effective) ways that are not covered by the approved label. This is called off label use. Most insurance carriers are not concerned with such use because they trust their participating doctors, but some insurance companies won't pay for off label drug use. This can severely limit a doctor's freedom to choose a chemotherapy treatment for you although of course it provides substantial savings for the insurance company. If this happens to you, alert your doctor or his or her business office, and then make use of your insurance company's appeals process.

- You may be using the drug as part of a clinical trial (see the section on breast cancer in chapter 4). Some insurance companies refuse to pay the costs for clinical trials because they think that investigative treatment may not be effective. Yet these treatments are often very effective and are indispensable to cancer research. Almost everything we know about cancer has come from the use of clinical trials. Limiting their use will slow our progress toward finding more cures for cancer.

It is always possible, of course, that your doctor may be using a drug or therapy that is unsafe or ineffective. See chapter 8 for a discussion of unsafe and ineffective cancer treatments.

What If You Don't Have Insurance?

For almost thirty million Americans, most of this chapter is academic and of little practical value because they have no insurance.

Many of these people work full time but fall into the gap between government programs and private health insurance. They make too much money to qualify for Medicaid, are too young for Medicare, are too healthy for the Medicare disability plan, and don't make enough to afford a private health insurance policy.

Others have had some prior illness that disqualifies them from affordable insurance. Some have changed jobs or become unemployed and lost coverage. Some can't get insurance because of some high-risk behavior, such as smoking or alcoholism. And there are always a few who can get insurance but don't, either through laziness or the presumption that they won't need it.

If you are one of these gap people, you are among the growing number of Americans who face financial devastation from a major illness like cancer.

What can you do if you are diagnosed with cancer and fall into this situation? We suggest that you ask for direction and help from the Cancer Information Service at the National Cancer Institute. You can also call the American Cancer Society, the Leukemia Society of America, the National Coalition of Cancer Survivors, or other organizations whose addresses and phone numbers are listed in the appendix. Many of these organizations have information pamphlets, available through your local cancer center, that can be of help. In addition, although these organizations may not be able to provide large sums of money to provide for treatment, they often have enough to help with expenses for travel, pain medications, and some doctor bills in certain situations. Your community may have a free clinic that you can start out with. Many nonprofit hospitals also have a teaching service, where patients are accepted regardless of their ability to pay. Some people without insurance have resorted to mass appeals, using mass media (radio, television, or newspapers) to raise funds. Others have told their churches of their situations, and churches have organized benefits and taken offerings to help. In our own community, there have been many successful fund drives to help pay for expensive medical care. These drives have been particularly effective for children or young parents who have cancer or other serious illnesses. Even in times of economic recession, people seem to open their purses when their heartstrings are tugged.

Whatever you do, don't let worry about finances keep you from seeking medical help for your symptoms. Unfortunately, many people without insurance delay visits to the doctor until the cancer is far advanced. At that point, the cancer may be far more expensive to treat and the outcome less favorable.

This chapter has attempted to prepare you to face the often troubling financial concerns that usually accompany a diagnosis of cancer. We hope it has helped allay your fears or at least reduced the fear of the unknown. If you still have questions, we suggest that you check with your doctor's office manager or the business office of your hospital for people who can help answer your questions.

8

What about Coffee Enemas?

Recognizing False Promises—
Medical and Spiritual

Charlie was a surgeon in his early fifties who learned he had cancer of the bladder. The recommended treatment was surgery, and with this treatment the prognosis was quite good—but the surgery would leave him impotent, without his bladder, and requiring an external drainage apparatus. Charlie panicked at the prospect of such unpleasant side effects. Instead of making plans for his operation, he flew to the Bahamas for immunoaugmentative therapy.

After six months of this treatment, however, Charlie felt even worse, so he returned home and agreed to the surgery. But it was too late. His cancer had spread to the point where surgery would be useless and his survival unlikely. Six months of unconventional (and ineffective) treatment in the Bahamas had allowed his cancer to progress past the point of no return.[1]

Immunoaugmentative therapy is just one of many unproven and sometimes dangerous "alternative" (*p. 154) treatments that promise to cure cancer. Every year, thousands of cancer patients, like Charlie,

incur grave danger and sometimes forfeit cures from traditional treatments because they are persuaded that an unconventional treatment
could be their salvation.

This chapter will describe the unproven (and suspect) treatments to
which cancer patients in this country most commonly subscribe and
will attempt to point out the dangers of each one. At the end of the
chapter is a checklist of questions you may want to ask when evaluating nontraditional therapies. We hope our analysis will help protect
you or your loved ones from spending thousands of dollars and hours
chasing a cure that may do nothing more than fill someone's bank
account. But first, let's take a closer look at who typically tries these
unconventional methods—and why.

Who Uses These Treatments?

Unproven, unconventional cancer treatment is big business in the
United States. The late Congressman Claude Pepper's Select Sub-
committee on Quackery determined that more than ten billion dollars
is spent annually by people who bypass traditional medicine seeking
cures for cancer. This is hardly surprising. Traditional medicine does
not pretend to have all the answers for cancer patients; it concedes that
many of those who receive the best treatment die. Cancer patients,
especially those who believe their cancer is terminal, are naturally
drawn to any method that guarantees success.

It's a mistake to assume that only uneducated, naive people would
spend their money and time on unproven methods of treatment. In
fact, the surgeon mentioned above is not unusual. Most of those
drawn to unconventional methods are intelligent, educated people.
Studies by Barrie Cassileth at the University of Pennsylvania Cancer
Center indicate that the average patient who seeks unorthodox treatment is well educated and in an early stage of cancer.[2]

Gregory A. Curt, M.D., of the Clinical Oncology Program at the
National Cancer Institute concurs with this finding: "Often it's the

---

*By alternative treatment, we mean nontraditional therapies that are unproven and
used outside the setting of a clinical trial.

highly motivated, highly educated, successful patient with early stage disease, curable by surgery, who is attracted to alternative therapies."[3]

Many who are drawn to alternative treatments are movers and shakers who have beaten the odds before, either in business or relationships. They are used to rolling up their shirtsleeves to attack problems aggressively. Since this strategy has worked before in other areas of their lives, they believe it can work again to solve their physical problems.

Those who turn to alternative methods of treatment also tend to be relatively well-to-do. The reason for this is simple. It is usually only people with money who can afford to travel to distant clinics, purchase special equipment and foods, and make a major commitment of time and energy. Even the British royal family uses and supports alternative medicine. In 1983, Prince Charles made a well-publicized trip to Bristol to open a cancer help center that specializes in complementary methods of treatment. Alternative medicine is one of the few growth industries in contemporary Britain.

Most practitioners of these alternative methods are not what we would normally call quacks. A majority are trained physicians who simply ignore the regulatory guidelines established by the Food and Drug Administration. Many are sincerely trying to help patients but are misled by dubious claims of scientific validity. Others may be seeking financial gain.

Why Are People Drawn to Alternative Therapies?

Why are educated people so willing to spend huge sums of money and time on methods that are questionable at best? There are several answers to this question. The first, and simplest, lies in human nature. When given a choice between the pleasant and the unpleasant, we gravitate toward the pleasant. And when offered a conventional treatment that may well be unpleasant and holds no guarantees, we are naturally attracted to a doctor or a program that offers the moon.

A Distrust of Traditional Medicine

Another reason so many people find alternative treatments appealing is that many distrust the medical profession in general and conventional cancer therapy in particular. They may even have seen friends or family suffer bad side effects from radiation or chemotherapy and then die. So they may wrongly assume that the chemo or the radiation caused the deaths and therefore decide to steer away from such treatments. They become determined to look elsewhere for help when confronted with the worst sickness of their lives.

Some of Bill's patients are afraid of traditional medical treatments because they only have experience with now-outdated methods of surgery and radiation. "Uncle Harry took that cobalt treatment in the 1950s," one man told him, "and it burnt him up! No way am I going to take that radiation!" Such an unpleasant memory is indeed a powerful reason to avoid traditional therapy. But because of the tremendous advances made in radiation therapy, it is also a very bad reason.

Some people are turned off by what they perceive as a clinical, uncaring attitude on the part of doctors and hospitals. Unfortunately, some of this reputation is deserved. For instance, while some oncologists (cancer specialists) are warm and empathetic, the specialty as taught in medical schools tends to foster a rather cool, detached approach. This cool professionalism will often get the job done, but it can also send a message (usually unintended) that the doctors don't really care. Patients may feel their doctors think of them as tumors or conditions instead of as people. Many hospitals, too, can seem cold, uncaring—designed to process patients instead of healing people.

Alternative medicine, on the other hand, typically boasts, "We care!" Pamphlets show pastoral settings, warm hugs, and smiling faces. They talk about treating the whole person. For patients who need emotional as much as physical comfort, this approach is enormously appealing. (This aspect of nontraditional treatments is one we believe the conventional medical community would do well to learn from.)

Some people also turn from the traditional medical channels because they simply don't understand how cancer works. They may have read literature claiming that an unhealthy lifestyle causes cancer. If bad diet and lifestyle cause cancer, they figure, then proper diet and lifestyle can cure it. Such a simplistic understanding could make a person an easy target for unrealistic claims from nontraditional practitioners.

Patterns in American Culture

Cassileth and his colleague Deborah Berlyne are convinced that certain patterns in American culture contribute to the popularity of alternative medicine. The first is our confidence in the ability of the rugged individual to beat great odds. From the frontiersman of early America to John Wayne and Rambo, Americans have admired and tried to emulate those individuals who defy convention and strike out on their own, against great odds, to pursue their dreams or conquer evil. Cassileth and Berlyne maintain that we believe we can do the same if we just imitate our heroes' strength of resolve.[4]

We also tend, they argue, to invent a cause for a problem if the cause is not known. So if traditional medicine says it does not know the cause of some cancers, we have little trouble believing those practitioners who proclaim they have scientifically found the source of cancer—whether it be constipation, protein metabolism malfunction, or "caustic soda irritation of body cells."[5]

According to Cassileth, this is not the first time that Americans have given up on traditional medicine and sought out unorthodox solutions. The nineteenth century, known by some medical historians as the golden age of quackery, produced many self-care cults, and much of their rhetoric has a familiar ring to it.

For example, many groups then criticized the medical profession for taking the responsibility for health out of the hands of the patient. They called for the democratization of medical knowledge, with "every man his own doctor." What was needed, they cried, was a "holistic" self-care alternative to a disease-oriented, impersonal medical system. The gospel of today's "medical counter-culture" (Cassileth's phrase) is much the same.

What one observer wrote in 1932 illustrates why alternative cancer cures are so popular today: The patient feels "that there is no one who really sees him or is interested in him as a whole. The cults have capitalized on this failure of modern medicine to view the patient as an entity, and [modern medicine's mistake of replacing] the old family physician with a coordinated specialism."[6] If this was true in 1932, how much more true is it today?

Promises, Promises: Common Unconventional Treatments

Nontraditional treatments that promise cures for cancer come from several channels today. In the pages to come, we will examine some of the most popular.

"If You Only Believe"—The Radical Faith Healers

Probably the best-known nontraditional cancer remedy is popularly called faith healing. It is based on the premise that God will heal any sick person who "truly believes" in this healing.

Now, we are not saying that cancer is never healed by divine intervention. We are both Christians who believe strongly in God's sovereign power. And as we will argue in chapter 13, we believe that physical healing by the power of God is still possible today. At the same time, we recommend that faith in God for healing always be accompanied by the best of what traditional medicine has to offer.

Some practitioners of faith healing, on the other hand, reject all reliance on traditional medicine as unspiritual, symptomatic of unbelief. In the process, we believe, they not only distort the Word of God, but they also endanger the very people who trust them.

Let's look a bit more closely at the claims of radical faith healers. God is obligated to heal you, they preach, if you make a confession of faith. God has stated in the Bible that he will do for you whatever you truly believe. So if you truly believe that God will heal you, he is bound by his Word to cure your disease.

Confession of the mouth is usually a key term for those who advocate this approach. What you say with your lips (the confession of the mouth) determines what happens to you. If you confess prosperity and health, you will experience prosperity and health. But if you confess poverty or sickness, you will experience the same. A negative confession, they warn, will produce sickness. If you tell someone that you think you are getting sick, then you probably will; words have power to bring things into being. In fact, a negative confession of sickness is believed to give Satan the right to inflict a person with sickness.

The notion that negative confession produces sickness goes even further. E. W. Kenyon (1867–1948), a Christian pastor and radio preacher who directly influenced today's radical faith healers, taught that to talk about illness is tantamount to devil worship and can even infect others with illness.

The consequences of this teaching can be seen in some "faith" churches that rebuke those who talk of illness, telling them instead to confess the Word and give thanks for their healing. In such churches, symptoms of illness are denied. Symptoms are viewed as spiritual smoke screens through which Satan tricks believers into making negative confessions, thus forfeiting their healings.

As Kenneth Hagin, the most prominent radical faith healer today, has written, "Real faith in God—heart faith—believes the Word of God regardless of what the physical evidences may be. . . . A person seeking healing should look to God's Word, not to his symptoms."[7]

Hagin brazenly declares, moreover, that it is always God's will to heal cancer.

> I believe that it is the plan of God our Father that no believer should ever be sick. That every believer should live his full length of time and actually wear out, if Jesus tarries, and fall asleep in Jesus. It is not—I state boldly—it is not the will of God my Father that we should suffer with cancer and other dread diseases which bring pain and anguish. No! It is God's will that we be healed.[8]

Fred Price, another leader in this movement, describes a situation in which he was determined not to confess sickness despite great pain.

> I have been attacked to such a degree, and been in such pain that I almost wished that I had never heard about faith and healing. Sometimes I would hurt so badly until I wanted to go to the doctors and let

them give me a shot, and knock me out for six weeks, and that would have been easy. But I knew better. . . . I refused to give in to it.[9]

As is evident, Price and others teach that medicine only helps relieve the pain and symptoms of the illness; it is incapable of attacking the illness itself. Because all sickness is spiritual rather than physical in origin, only spiritual weapons are of any avail. Those who resort to medicine, therefore, are fools to use a physical weapon to attack a spiritual problem.

"Doctors are fighting the same enemies that we are," Price explains. "The only difference is they're using toothpicks and we are using atomic bombs." Hence only the immature believer will rely on such a crutch as medicine: "If you need a crutch or something to help you get along, then praise God, hobble along until you get your faith moving to the point that you don't need a crutch."[10]

What happens to people who try to put the ideas of radical faith healers into practice? Some claim that it works for them; they insist they have been healed. But those who are not healed—and this may be a majority—probably feel guilt and condemnation. For if Hagin and Price are right, failure to experience healing is always the fault of the believer.

Price clearly implies, for instance, that anyone who dies before the age of seventy and dies of anything but old age has missed God's will, either because of sin or unbelief.

Your minimum days should be 70 years, that's just the bare minimum. You ought to live to be at least 120 years of age. That's the Bible. God out of his own mouth—in the Old Testament—said the number of your days shall be 120 years. I didn't write it! God said it. The minimum ought to be 70 years, and you shouldn't go out with sickness and disease then.[11]

Besides filling cancer patients with guilt and condemnation for their failure to find healing, radical faith teachers send some people to the grave far sooner than necessary. Since use of medicine and doctors is considered unspiritual and even sinful, many followers of these teachers have shunned treatment even when afflicted with treatable life-threatening illness. The result has often been tragic.

Hobart Freeman was the pastor of Faith Assembly in Wilmot, Indiana, from 1978 to 1984. According to a story in the 2 June 1984 edition of the *Fort Wayne News Sentinel*, estimates of the number of preventable deaths associated with Faith Assembly alone run as high as ninety.[12] Several physicians in Tulsa, Oklahoma (Hagin's base of operations), have told D. R. McConnell, a historian of the modern faith movement, that patients often come to them too late because they deny their symptoms. One cancer specialist lamented that he sees such people every week, and that in many cases this denial made a significant difference in their chances of recovery.[13]

As chapter 13 will show, this teaching of radical faith healers has support in neither the Bible nor Christian theology. This is ironic, of course, because radical faith teachers appeal to the Bible to support their doctrine that God always wants to heal every illness. Yet, as we will see, both Paul and Timothy had illnesses from which they were not healed, and Jesus chose to heal some people but not others.

Paul wrote in Romans 8 that all of creation groans under the curse of suffering and won't be released from the curse till the end of the world. Believers, too, he wrote, await the "redemption of their bodies."[14] If the Bible really teaches that God intends all believers to be free of disease, why does it say that suffering will remain and that our bodies won't be redeemed until the end? Hagin, Price, and their brethren talk as if the body can be redeemed now if only we have enough faith. We believe this approach is both unfounded and harmful.

Mind over Matter: The Simontons and Bernie Siegel

A second very common alternative approach to healing is that taken by O. Carl Simonton, Stephanie Matthews-Simonton, and Bernie Siegel.[15] All three are physicians who recommend therapy that is psychological rather than religious or spiritual. Like the faith healers, they make claims that have not been proven clinically.

Siegel, for instance, claims that cancer is psychosomatic in origin — that it originates in the patient's mind. Though he has some evidence from his own practice that some of his patients' cancers were affected by their attitudes, he can offer no proof that there is a similar connection for all other people who suffer from cancer.

These alternative treatments, therefore, pose similar risks to those offered by radical faith healers. Patients may avoid traditional treatment (although both the Simontons and Siegel generally recommend the use of traditional therapies as well) and may suffer from terrible guilt and condemnation if their cancers are not healed. For, like the radical faith healers, these therapies imply (and Siegel sometimes states explicitly) that cancer is the patient's own fault.

In one respect, however, the Simonton-Siegel approach is fundamentally different from the faith healers' strategy. The Simontons and Siegel proclaim that the human self has all the power it needs to cure cancer, while the faith healers point to a being outside themselves as the ultimate source of healing. In other words, Siegel and the Simontons argue that we can heal ourselves of cancer by tapping into our inner energies, while the faith healers — and the Christian faith for that matter — insist that God is the primary healer of the human soul or body.

Carl Simonton was originally trained in radiation oncology but then began to teach the importance of relaxation and imagery for curing cancer. In 1975, he and Stephanie Matthews-Simonton published an article in the *Journal of Transpersonal Psychology* that described a study of 152 patients' attitudes after they had received radiotherapy. According to the article, those who improved after treatment had a positive outlook, while those whose condition continued to deteriorate tended to be pessimistic. There was no way to know with certainty whether the radiotherapy influenced these patients' attitudes or whether the patients' attitudes caused their recovery or deterioration. But the Simontons chose to believe the latter.

From that point on, the Simontons' message proved to be enormously popular. Their book, *Getting Well Again: A Step-by-Step Self-Help Guide to Overcoming Cancer for Patients and Their Families*,[16] has been reprinted in more than twenty editions. Their Cancer Counseling and Research Center (now the Simonton Cancer Center) in Fort Worth, Texas, employs more than four thousand counselors and puts out a series of audiotape cassettes.

Bernie Siegel is an oncologist and surgeon in New Haven, Connecticut, and has taught at Yale University. He claims that the Simontons inspired him to explore the psychosomatic dimensions of cancer, and he published the results of his explorations in *Love, Medicine and Miracles: Lessons Learned about Self-Healing from a Surgeon's Experience with Exceptional Patients.*[17] It quickly became a bestseller.

Both Siegel and the Simontons teach that the secret of cancer is locked in the human mind. Cancer is both caused and cured, they argue, by human attitudes. For Siegel, cancer is simply depression expressed at the cellular level. It results from a failure to appropriate the "inner energy available to all of us . . . the life wish within . . . the mind's power."[18]

What this means, according to Siegel, is that healing is up to the individual, and it happens through hard work, not divine intervention. Those who have cancer must marshal the power of the mind to heal their bodies, for the condition of the body is the direct result of the state of the mind. In Siegel's words:

> The state of the mind changes the state of the body by working through the central nervous system, the endocrine system, and the immune system. Peace of mind sends the body a "live" message, while depression, fear and unresolved conflict give it a "die" message.[19]

What are we to make of the Simonton-Siegel approach? We cannot dismiss it out of hand, for thousands of people insist they have gained strength, peace, and even healing from one of the two therapies. And indeed, there is much to be said in favor of some aspects of these programs. The American Cancer Society, for example, has commended the Simontons' program on three counts: (1) it gives the patient a sense of control, (2) it promotes relaxation and well-being, (3) it causes no known deleterious effects.

And we can see four elements of Siegel's approach that are worthy of praise. First, Siegel rightly condemns our tendency to submit passively to the tyranny of the medical establishment. He champions the right of the patient to question the doctor's diagnosis and treatment. We agree that the patient has a far larger role to play in recovery than most of us have ever suspected. Patients, who often know their own bodies far better than physicians with all their technology can know, should therefore take an active, aggressive role in the struggle for healing.

Second, Siegel humbly admits that medical science does not have all the answers and cannot explain some healings that take place. Now, religious people have been saying this for centuries, but it is remarkable that this should come from the lips of a practicing oncologist who has taught at one of the nation's most prestigious universities. Our society tends to place too much faith in the power of medicine to cure the body's ills. Siegel and the religious traditions may disagree over where healing comes from, but they agree that it often does not come from medicine alone.

Third, Siegel is right, to a point, when he claims a connection between the attitudes of the mind and the condition of the body. The Western religious traditions have been saying the same thing for millennia. For instance, the author of the biblical Proverbs wrote more than 2,500 years ago,

> Do not be wise in your own eyes;
> fear the LORD and shun evil.
> This will bring health to your body
> and nourishment to your bones.[20]

So when Siegel writes that love, forgiveness, and the will to live are related to one's ability to survive cancer, he is echoing themes that Jews and Christians have affirmed for multiplied generations and that have been supported by many lifetimes of experience.

Finally, Siegel properly admonishes his fellow oncologists that they should be warm, open, and loving to their patients. He warns that they should reject the model the profession often encourages—

that of a cool, dispassionate expert who stays at arm's distance from his patients. Siegel hugs his patients and tries to show love to them.

For all of these reasons, we find much to applaud in Siegel's program. In fact, we wish that more oncologists would read his books because of the model of openness and compassion they portray. But we also have some grave concerns regarding both Siegel and the Simontons, and we wish that more patients and their friends would become aware of these concerns.

First, we are concerned that their basic premise—that the mind is always the final cause of the body's health or illness—is unproven. Studies have indeed suggested some relationship between attitudes and health, but the correlation is not nearly as strong as Siegel and the Simontons claim. There is no proof that negative attitudes cause cancer, nor is there proof that a positive attitude will cure cancer. As we said in chapter 2, if these assertions were true, psychiatric hospitals would be full of cancer patients, and cancer wards would be full of depressed people. Neither of these is true.

In fact, there is considerable research data pointing in the other direction.[21] D. K. Wellisch and J. Yager, for instance, closely examined studies linking depression and disease and concluded that these studies were poorly designed, used inaccurate personality measurements, displayed inherent selection bias, and were statistically imprecise.

S. Green and J. Maris, in an article in a 1975 issue of the *Journal of Psychometric Research*, reported on research that showed there was no correlation between attitude and the development of breast cancer. Three years later, a team of scientists issued the results of a long-term follow-up of World War II veterans who had been discharged because of "psychoneuroses." These veterans showed no increase in cancer when compared with a control group. In the same year, T. Niani and J. Jaaskleainen published the results of a twenty-two-year study of chronically depressed patients. The study revealed that these patients had the same rate of cancer as a control group without a history of depression.

A 1984 study published in the *New England Journal of Medicine* demonstrated that attitude seems to have no impact on the time-to-recurrence or survival of patients with advanced breast cancer or melanoma. B. H. Fox even argued in the *Journal of Psychosocial Oncology* that animal studies suggest stress can protect animals from developing cancer and retard the growth of implanted experimental tumors.

All of these studies fly in the face of the theory that attitude is both the universal cause and cure of cancer. There may be some people for whom attitude is a significant factor in the onset of cancer and others for whom attitude plays some role in their healing. But to claim that attitude is always the primary factor is simply to make a leap of faith—an unjustified one, in our opinion.

Even the medical experts in Bill Moyers's celebrated PBS series "Healing and the Mind" do not go that far. Not that they haven't found connections between mind and body. Dr. Pennebaker at Southern Methodist University discovered that when students wrote about traumatic events, one function in their immune systems was enhanced.[22] David and Suzanne Felten at the University of Rochester Medical School have discovered nerve fibers that link the nervous system and the immune system. Apparently the brain and the immune system talk to each other, which suggests a connection between our attitudes and our physical health.[23] Lydia Temoshek found that patients who expressed their feelings had more immune activity at the site of their lesions than those who were more reticent.[24]

But these researchers were careful not to claim that there is a direct relationship of cause and effect between certain attitudes and corresponding diseases. And they were even more cautious about asserting that thinking a certain way can guarantee healing. According to Robert Ader, director of behavioral and psychosocial medicine at the University of Rochester School of Medicine, "There are all kinds of advertisements for interventions to enhance your immune function and protect you against disease. These interventions may be based on reasonable hypotheses, but there are no data whatsoever to support these claims."[25] So while it is clear that spiritual and emotional wholeness can promote healing, there is no guarantee. We cannot say with any medical certainty that the mind can heal the body or that the mind alone causes cancer.

We also find the mind-over-matter theory suspect on theological grounds. The Jewish and Christian traditions have always taught that we are created in God's image and therefore have something of God's life within us. If we are healed, therefore, the healing is not necessarily coming from outside of us but from a Being who may be closer to us than our very bodies.

At the same time, both the Old and New Testaments teach that we cannot finally save or heal ourselves. The human body may have some natural curative powers, but they were put there by God. And those powers must be activated by God. To think that willpower or the human mind is the primary agent of healing borders on idolatry; it comes close to saying that we are divine.

The Bible teaches that we are not God, but God's, and that we reflect his nature as a mirror reflects the sun. Just as he thinks, feels, and acts, so do we. Just as his nature is moral, so is ours. But we are not omnipotent, omniscient, or omnipresent, as he is. Instead, we are finite and limited. He is sinless, but we are sinful. He is the Creator; we are created beings. To say that the creature has infinite capacities for healing is to claim divine power for what is less than divine. The Bible repeatedly condemns such human pretension to the divine throne.[26]

A final problem with Siegel's approach is that, like radical faith healers, it blames the patient for his or her cancer. At the very time when the cancer patient needs love and support—after healing has been sought but doesn't come—Siegel's book leaves the patient with guilt and condemnation. "There are no incurable diseases," he writes in *Love, Medicine and Miracles*, "only incurable people."[27] Whose fault is it, then, that healing didn't come? The implied answer is clear: the patient's!

"Years of experience have taught me that cancer and indeed nearly all diseases are psychosomatic."[28] Imagine telling that to a ten-year-old boy who is suffering with leukemia. How do you explain to him that he has brought on his own cancer by his bad attitude?

"I suggest that patients think of illness not as God's will but as our deviation from God's will. To me it is the absence of spirituality that leads to difficulties."[29] How do you say that to a woman who has tried to serve God all of her life? Do you tell her that her lack of devotion has filled her body with cancer? Can we really believe this?

"I feel that all disease is ultimately related to a lack of love, or to love that is only conditional, for the exhaustion and depression of the immune system thus created leads to physical vulnerability."[30] How does that explain the mean-spirited Scrooge who lives at the end of the block, tormenting his family and neighbors till the ripe old age of ninety? If lack of love always produces disease, he should have died long before.

Siegel did some backpedaling in his second book, *Peace, Love & Healing—Bodymind Communication & the Path to Self-Healing: An Exploration*.[31] In response to criticism for the guilt that his first book inspired, he wrote that illness and death should not be considered failures, that not every illness can be cured, that some things like the outcome of disease should be left up to God, and that death can be a healing and even a birth into eternal life.

Siegel never actually retracted the statements from his first book. Instead, he insisted that he had been misunderstood. Yet the concessions in his second book directly contradict the bold proclamations of the first book that there are no incurable diseases, that illness is a deviation from God's will and related to a lack of love, and that nearly all diseases are psychosomatic. Siegel has denied equating death with failure, but the unrepentant assertions of his first book and his mind-over-matter thesis continued in the second book both clearly imply it.

For these reasons, Bernie Siegel's program does not work for us. His approach can be helpful in that it teaches doctors to be open and compassionate. It has enlightened many cancer sufferers to their own important role in their treatment and recovery. And it accurately points out that sometimes healing has been promoted by attitudes of love, forgiveness, and the will to live. But its uncorrected generalization that cancer is caused by a failure to love and its continued implication that the person who dies from cancer has probably failed are both wrong and cruel. We agree with Ronni Sandroff, who writes, "It's bad enough that so many of our cancer patients do eventually die of their disease. But it seems a cruel addition not to challenge the belief that somehow it's their own . . . fault."[32]

Healing from a Peach Pit: Laetrile

In the 1960s and 1970s, when drugs were gaining increased acceptance as a legitimate treatment for cancer, laetrile was used on thousands of patients. The principal component of this drug is the compound amygdalin, which can be extracted from such natural sources as the pits of apricots, cherries, pears, apples, or peaches.[33]

In those first two decades of use, laetrile was administered without accurate readings of patient response or the drug's toxicity (potential to be poisonous). But in the last decade or so, careful studies have indicated not only that laetrile does not help fight cancer, but also that the treatment may be harmful.

The California Cancer Commission, for instance, found no responses in forty-four patients with a broad range of tumors who were treated with laetrile. A similar study by the National Cancer Institute followed 178 patients with a variety of cancers who were given laetrile. None of them showed improvement after treatment.

Ten Thousand and a Tune-Up—
Immunoaugmentative Therapy

In 1977, Dr. Lawrence Burton established his Immunology Researching Center in Freeport, Bahamas—after the FDA refused to allow its establishment in the United States. Dr. Burton bases his "immunoaugmentative therapy" (IAT) on the premise that cancer is caused by a deficiency of the immune system and that the remedy is to restore the immune system to health. His prescription is several weeks of injections of "immune serum protein fractions" at his center in the Bahamas—at a cost of ten thousand dollars—plus several "tune-ups" later. Thousands of Americans have taken Dr. Burton's treatments despite serious doubts regarding the effectiveness and safety of the treatments.

The Pan American Health Organization has recommended that the center be closed because of absence of any clinical evidence of its effectiveness. An independent analysis of the IAT serum fractions (the liquids that are injected into the patients) showed that they did not contain the blocking proteins, deblocking proteins, tumor antibodies, and tumor complements claimed by Dr. Burton. Instead, they are simple dilutions of blood plasma—nothing more than the liquid part of the blood, without red or white blood cells.

Even more ominous is the evidence that some of these blood-derived liquids have been tainted with the AIDS virus. The center has treated AIDS patients since the early 1980s. Apparently blood specimens from AIDS patients were mixed with blood specimens used to prepare treatments to be injected into cancer patients. An analysis of seventy-two vials of treatment materials available to the National Cancer Institute (NCI) showed that thirty-seven (51 percent) contained antibodies to HIV (the AIDS virus)—a strong indication that people injected with these materials could contract AIDS. And technicians at NCI were able to derive the AIDS virus from Dr. Burton's tainted treatment materials.

IAT, then, was an extremely dangerous treatment. Because of these findings, the clinic was closed in 1985, but it reopened after demonstrations in both Freeport and Washington. Testimonials from patients who claim benefit keep this and other clinics going.

"Get Back in Balance"—Metabolic Therapies

The premise of the last major group of unconventional therapies is that cancer is caused by an imbalance in the body's metabolism and that restoring the balance will cure cancer. There are many practitioners claiming many different ways of restoring metabolic balance. We will look at the five most common.

1. Dr. William Koch was a physician at the turn of the century who believed that cancer was a protective response to toxins (poisons) created by the body. To destroy these toxins, he prescribed enemas, a special diet, and his own antitoxin preparation, which was

essentially water (the label said it contained one part glyoxilide, a substance of dubious value, to one trillion parts water). The treatment was very popular when it first came out, and, amazingly, is still available today. There is no clinical evidence that it can fight cancer.

2. The International Health Institute, started by dentist William Kelly, proclaims that cancer is caused by a deficiency of pancreatic enzymes. The way to determine if you really have cancer, therefore, is to take six to eight pancreatic enzyme tablets after each meal for four weeks. At the end of this treatment, patients are told that if they feel worse, they probably have cancer. If they feel better, they have a precancerous condition. If they feel no different, they do not have cancer. All patients, both those who have cancer and those who want to prevent cancer, are told to follow a low-protein diet with mineral supplements, yogurt enemas, and induced sweating.

3. The East West Center for Macrobiotics and the Kushi Foundation are among the many diet-based programs that claim to cure cancer. Their particular approach to diet is based on the Chinese belief in yin and yang, two cosmic forces whose interactions are said to determine everything that happens in the universe. Cancers of the yin organs (colon, stomach, bladder) are treated with yang foods (fruit, fish, cooked vegetables), while cancers of yang organs (lungs, liver) are treated with yin foods (raw vegetables, no fruit, no fish). Foods that are prohibited include meat, dairy products, sweets, processed foods, and hot spices.

   This sort of diet is dangerous because, depending on the combination of foods, it can be deficient in calories, vitamins C and D, and/or iron. Both children and adults on this diet have shown nutritional deficiencies. Most important, there is no scientific evidence that this diet prevents or retards the growth of cancer.

4. Megavitamin therapy (also called orthomolecular treatment) is based on the premise that large doses of certain vitamins can assist

the immune system in its fight against foreign growths, including cancer. In particular, vitamin C is said to reduce tumor cell production of enzymes that invade new cells and spread cancer to other parts of the body.

Although an early study seemed to show improvement in patients given vitamin C, more controlled studies later showed no evidence that large doses of vitamins shrank tumors or helped patients felt better. They did compile considerable evidence, however, that large doses of some vitamins can have toxic effects.

Five to ten thousand units of vitamin A over thirty days, for example, has been shown to cause increased intracranial pressure, fetal abnormalities, and liver and kidney poisoning. Researchers have determined that vitamin E is ineffective by itself as a weapon against cancer and that high doses can cause significant health problems. In one study, six hundred units a day increased triglyceride levels in the blood, nine hundred per day caused depression and fatigue, while thirty-two hundred units per day caused nausea, diarrhea, headaches, and blurred vision. High doses in animals have lowered bone calcium and atrophied testicles.

A substance that some vitamin-therapy practitioners call vitamin B15 is perhaps the most alarming. It is not in fact a vitamin, but contains two compounds that are known to be carcinogens.

These studies do not seem to have stopped the growth of what amounts to a health fraud industry in this country. Practitioners of nutritional supplements can get degrees in nutrition by mail: one thousand dollars for a bachelor's degree, two thousand for both bachelor's and master's, four thousand for a bachelor's, master's, and doctor of philosophy.

5. Combined approaches are prescribed by some unconventional programs. Many combine diet with vitamins and detoxification, which is supposed to occur through wheat-grass therapy or coffee enemas. The theory behind coffee enemas is that exposure of the liver to caffeine will render harmless the impurities that have thrown the body's metabolism out of balance.

Two of the best-known programs that use a combined approach are run by Dr. Ernesto Contreras and Hans Nieper. Dr. Contreras operates the Centro Medico Del Mar of Tijuana, Mexico, where standard drugs and hormones are prescribed in addition to laetrile, cell therapy, interferons (a family of proteins closely linked to the immune system — see chapter 5), and enzyme enemas. At Mr. Nieper's clinic in Germany, patients receive chemotherapy plus vitamin A, anavit (a pineapple enzyme), shark-liver extract, Venus flytrap extract, laetrile, and mineral therapy.

What are we to make of these combined approaches? As you might have guessed, few of these therapies have been proven to be of any help against cancer. Many rely on anecdotal rather than scientific evidence. Some in fact may be toxic. If some patients are cured, it is probably because of the conventional therapies also used.

Caveat Emptor (Let the Buyer Beware)

This chapter has demonstrated that no cancer therapy, least of all unconventional and unproven ones, is without its harmful side effects. The radical faith healer and the Simonton-Siegel approaches can leave the patient no better off than when he or she started — and full of destructive guilt to boot. Many of the unorthodox medical therapies have been shown to be totally ineffective against cancer and some are even poisonous. But even if the treatment is harmless, a patient can waste money that could be better used for conventional, proven treatment. Worse still, a patient may put off life-saving treatment while seeking a cure by unorthodox means. Then, as for the surgeon described at the beginning of this chapter, it may be too late.

If you are considering a nontraditional, unproven therapy, try asking these questions before you sign on the dotted line:

- Is the approach scientific? What is the evidence that it will work? Has it been published in scientific journals? If not, why not?

- Who is promoting the therapy? Is it someone who stands to benefit personally?

- Do the promoters claim that you can certainly be healed if only you have enough faith or love?

- Do promoters forbid you to confess your symptoms?

- Do promoters claim that all disease has only one cause, or that their treatment is all that is needed to fight cancer?

- Do the claims for healing sound too good to be true? (They probably are.)

- Do the promoters make you alone or the power within ultimately responsible for your health?

- Is the primary proof from testimonials rather than from verifications by reputable health professionals?

- What will the treatment cost? Will your insurance cover it?

- Can you continue your regular treatments and try the unproven treatment at the same time?[34]

9

Why Me, God?

The Age-Old Problem of Evil—
And Some Answers We Can't Accept

Cancer is one of the most frightening and confusing words in the English language. If you or someone you love has cancer, you already know that.

Perhaps your heart started pounding after you first got the news. Or maybe it waited until you left the doctor's office or got off the phone. And whether you or a loved one has cancer, you have probably spent sleepless nights tormenting yourself with the question that has haunted men and women since the dawn of time—the question of why.

Floyd is asking that question. He is a thirty-three-year-old single parent whose three-year-old son, Jimmy, has just been diagnosed with leukemia. At this point, it looks as if Jimmy will live, and Jimmy seems to enjoy all the attention he is getting from doctors, nurses, and his family. But Floyd is beside himself; he fluctuates between terror and rage as the questions consume him. What will this illness do to the rest of Jimmy's life? Will he have a greater chance of getting cancer again in the future? Will the leukemia deprive him of a normal childhood?

And where is God in all of this? If he is really all-good and all-powerful, why does he allow such a terrible thing like cancer? This last question particularly torments Floyd.

In our own experience—personal and professional—we have discovered that there is no one answer to this most difficult of questions—no single answer that fits every situation. Instead, we have discovered a range of answers that, though different from one another, are all attested by both Scripture and good Christian theology. Each one has proven helpful to thousands of people, both in the past and more recently. For each answer there are thousands of people who can say, "This speaks to my experience! I know this is the best answer to my question about cancer!"

We will present these answers in chapters 10 and 11. But first we want to explore some popular answers that have also proven helpful to many but that, for reasons we will explain, we cannot accept.

Just a Chance Occurrence?

The first answer we cannot accept is that diseases such as cancer are simply the result of being human in this world.

According to this view, there is a God, but he is not in control of everything that happens. The basic processes of nature, for instance, operate independently of God's governance. Diseases are accidents that occur for no particular reason, other than the fact that nature is known statistically to produce countless defects.

Rabbi Harold Kushner, who offers this answer in *When Bad Things Happen to Good People*,[1] watched his son die at age fourteen from the rare disease progeria, which is characterized by an accelerated aging process. Such a death, he concluded, is simply bad luck, "an inevitable consequence of our being human and being mortal, living in a world of inflexible natural laws."

For Kushner, God is imperfect. He cannot protect human beings from such tragedies because the laws of nature are outside his control. It is therefore our responsibility to forgive and to love God despite his limitations. If we do that, we will find that he weeps with us in our sorrow and gives us the strength to carry on.

Now there is much to be said for Kushner's answer to this age-old problem of evil. While many use an experience like cancer to paint God as a harsh schoolmaster administering cruel and unusual punishments, Kushner insists that God is good. He does not enjoy torturing people with disease, Kushner rightly proclaims, but hates evil and unfairness.

In fact, the Bible portrays God as a loving heavenly Father who cares for his children tenderly and passionately.[2] Jesus said that God takes the initiative to forgive and restore his children when they have rebelled against him.[3] Such a God cares deeply about the suffering of human beings, even those who turn against him.[4]

Kushner is also correct when he says that God does not prevent calamities, but gives us strength and perseverance to endure them. Millions of readers have received comfort from his suggestion that God suffers with us and stands beside us when we suffer, and that he answers our prayers for strength, compassion, and courage.

So we applaud much of what Kushner has taught through his books. But we cannot accept his answer to the why question because that answer denies a central affirmation of our faith—that God controls this world.

The Bible portrays God as great and all-powerful,[5] the power above all other powers[6] who "makes clouds rise from the ends of the earth; he sends lightning with the rain and brings out the wind from his storehouses."[7] In other words, God is completely in control of the powers of nature. If cancer is a product of the forces of nature, then it cannot be outside of God's control.

Jesus said that apart from God not even a sparrow falls to the ground.[8] If that is true, how can cancer be totally unrelated to God's will? It may not be directly ordained by God, but Jesus implies that nothing (therefore not even cancer) is completely outside his control.

Part of a Fallen World?

Another popular answer to the question of why a good God would allow cancer is that this world is not as it should be. At one time the world was entirely good since it was created by a good God. But then something happened to bring evil into the world, and cancer is part of that evil. God is therefore only indirectly involved with the origin of cancer. He watches from a distance, as it were, as cancer springs up in the world.

Again we have to admit that there is much to commend this view. The Bible tells us that there was a fall when sin and death entered the world, and that since that time humanity and nature have been different. Because sin has so deeply affected the very fabric of existence, nothing is as it should be. It is no surprise that there are terrible diseases like cancer that distort the normal functioning of the human body.

This much we can accept. But we cannot accept the notion that God has nothing to do with the distortions of this fallen world. If God is all-powerful, he could intervene to stop evil. Sometimes it seems that he does just that. But many other times he permits evil to continue unchecked. Why? This is the question that faces us.

Punishment for Adam's Sin?

Some say that God permits evil in order to punish humanity for Adam's sin. Adam, they argue, was our representative before God. Therefore, the consequences of his actions have fallen upon his descendants. Since he chose to sin, we and the rest of the human race were given the penalty of living in a fallen world that would be filled with, among other things, deadly diseases such as cancer.

We see the same element of truth in this view that we saw in the previous view. Everyday experience tells us that this is indeed a fallen world, corrupted by sin. But to say that all evil, including cancer, is a punishment for Adam's sin contradicts the biblical portrait of God.

The biblical authors describe God as just—in fact, as the author and standard of all justice.[9] Is it just for God to punish us for something that someone else has done? The prophet Ezekiel didn't seem to think so: "The son will not share the guilt of the father."[10] Neither do we. Because this view agrees with neither the biblical portrait of God nor our own sense of fairness, we cannot accept it.[11]

The Work of Satan?

Another common answer is that evil in the world is simply the work of Satan. This world, it is said, is a battlefield between God and the devil, and evil reflects the latter's presence. Terrible things like cancer cannot possibly be part of God's will. They are from the Prince of Darkness who, for some mysterious reason, has been allowed by the God of Light to have the upper hand for a while.

This view can claim some support in the Bible and human experience. Scripture asserts that Satan is the "ruler of this world,"[12] and occasionally names him as the author of disease. Job, for example, is sent painful boils by Satan; Jesus says in Luke's Gospel that a crippled woman was a victim of Satan[13]; and Paul writes that a malady he called his "thorn in the flesh" was a messenger of Satan.[14]

Many of us have known times when we have sensed the vivid presence of evil—a force that goes beyond what even human sin can accomplish. Some time ago, when I (Gerry) was giving a lecture on Luther's view of the devil, an older woman with a German accent told the church audience that when she was a child in Nazi Germany, she and her family could feel an evil power at work in the land. "It was so thick," she recalled, "you could cut it with a knife. It was clear that this was not just the result of what people did, but that there was an evil force in the air."

We agree that the Bible does attribute some sickness to Satan. And our experience tells us that a real power of evil does seem to be at work in the world. But this answer, like the others, does not really respond to the question of why a good, all-powerful God would permit cancer. Even if cancer is the result of Satan's evil acts in the world, the question still remains: why does God continue to permit it? If God is all-powerful, he could prevent the outbreak and spread of cancer. Why doesn't he? Even those who attribute cancer to Satan admit that God somehow allows Satan temporary freedom to do his evil work. If Satan is like a dog on a leash, with freedom to do only as much as his Master allows, why does the divine Master allow him to afflict us with cancer?

So we are back to where we started. Why does God allow cancer? The popular answers today that either deny God's involvement in cancer (cancer is just a chance occurrence) or say that he is only indirectly involved (cancer is punishment for Adam's sin or the work of Satan) do not do justice to the biblical insistence that God is in control of this world. Let's turn, then, to other answers that we think do a better job of responding to the question, "Why does God allow cancer?"

10

Is Cancer
Part of God's Plan?

*Some Promising Answers to
the Age-Old Question*

We read in the last chapter about Floyd, the single parent whose three-year-old son, Jimmy, has been diagnosed with leukemia. Though Jimmy does not fully understand the dangers of this cancer, Floyd does. Right now, therefore, Floyd is the one who's really suffering. And the question that is tormenting Floyd is the same question that millions of believers have asked for centuries: If God is all-good and all-powerful, why would he permit a terrible disease like cancer?

Floyd's neighbor John, an insurance salesman, came over one evening to try to comfort Floyd. After making small talk in Floyd's kitchen, John said, "Floyd, if there's any way that I can help, please let me know. Even if you just need someone to talk to."

"That's exactly what I need, John. You know, right now Jimmy isn't in any pain, so he's not really suffering. And I'm not worried about the financial end of things; I've got pretty good insurance. But what I can't stop thinking about is the justice of it all."

"What do you mean?" John asked.

"Well, I've been going to church every week since Mary and I divorced. So I've been trying, in my own way, to come back to God. And now, what do I get? Jimmy comes down with cancer!"

John was not a churchgoer himself. He had been raised in a fundamentalist church that preached hellfire and brimstone. Turned off as a teenager, he had left the church with the general impression that God is full of vengeance and punishes people for their sins.

"Floyd, I'm probably not the right person to talk to. I really don't know what to think about God. But sometimes I think bad things happen to me because God is punishing me for not going to church. Other times I don't. So who knows? Maybe you've sinned, and this is your punishment."

God's Punishment for an Individual's Sin?

We have found that a surprising number of people, either consciously or unconsciously, subscribe to this notion that cancer may be a punishment from God for past sins. One of Bill's patients, for instance, was convinced that her breast cancer was a punishment for having had an abortion some years earlier. Another, a seventy-year-old man, believed his prostate cancer was a punishment for having rebelled against his father, who also had suffered from prostate cancer.

Now, it is true that some parts of the Bible do seem to point to a connection between human wrongdoing and human suffering. For instance, the Old Testament God does sometimes send suffering as punishment for sin. The flood wiped out Noah's generation because of their wickedness. When the Israelites in the wilderness complained about a lack of water and decent food, God sent poisonous snakes to wreak havoc among the people. The Old Testament prophets proclaimed that Israel's defeats and exiles were God's chastening for its idolatry. Even Jesus hinted at a possible connection between sin and suffering when he healed a man who had been sick for thirty-eight years. He declared, "See, you are well again. Stop sinning or something worse may happen to you."[1]

Experience, too, does point to a limited connection between some sinful behavior and certain diseases. A person who is sexually promis-cuous, for example, is certainly at risk for venereal disease or AIDS, and we saw in chapter 2 that at least one type of cancer (cervical can-cer) is associated with sexual promiscuity. Smoking, which could be seen as a sin against the body, is also strongly associated with several diseases, especially lung cancer.

God Doesn't Usually Work That Way

But this suggestion of a cause-and-effect relationship quickly breaks down when we view the whole of the biblical message and the entirety of experience. For every case in which a clear connection between sin and suffering can be made, we have even clearer examples of instances where the suffering did not result from sin.

The Bible, in fact, depicts several instances in which those people who assume that suffering is a punishment for sin are directly rebuked. For example, there is the case of the man born blind, whose story is told in the Gospel of John. Jesus' disciples asked if the blindness was a result of the man's sin or his parents' sin. Jesus replied categorically that neither had been responsible: "He is blind so that God's power might be seen at work in him."[2]

The biblical story of Job is another powerful example of suffering that is clearly not the result of sin. At the beginning of the story, we are told clearly that Job's afflictions have come not because of any fault of Job's but because of a cosmic argument between God and Satan. And Job's comforters, who try to argue that Job's suffering is the result of sin, are roundly refuted.

Then there are the Galileans who were executed by Pilate and the eighteen Jews who were killed when the Tower of Siloam fell on them. Jesus' disciples asked him if these people suffered because they were worse sinners than their neighbors. In both cases, Jesus emphat-ically replied, "No!"[3]

In personal experience, too, we have known many wonderful people struck by terrible illness and mean-spirited never-do-wells who have lived long, healthy lives. Floyd's small son, for instance, was simply not old enough to "deserve" the painful punishment of leukemia. What three-year-old is? And God doesn't punish the child for the sins of its parent.

We are convinced, therefore, that except in certain very special cases, there is no cause-and-effect relationship between sin and cancer. In the vast majority of cases, God just does not work that way. He is a God of great compassion and love. He loves us even when we don't love him. As Jesus said, he came not to condemn but to save.[4] You and I would be presumptuous and probably cruelly wrong to assume that someone else's cancer is a result of her or his sin or even that our own cancer is the result of our own sin.

More to the point, there are other answers that are more compatible with Scripture and with the experience of thousands of people who have said, "Yes! This answer perfectly describes my situation!"

It May Take a While to Sort It Out

Before we outline these answers, however, let us comment on their applicability. It has been our experience that cancer patients and their families, even those with deep faith, often remain confused and disturbed while they are experiencing the trauma of cancer about why God allowed this to come to them. This may be true for you, as well.

If you or someone you love is currently undergoing cancer treatment, you may not be able to affirm any of the answers we present. It may not be until much later, after you have gone through the experience of cancer and have had time to recover and reflect, that you will be able to come to any sort of clarity about why all this has occurred. It is possible that even after years have passed you will still find yourself wrestling with these issues. These are hard questions—questions that human beings have struggled with since the dawn of time. They cannot be honestly resolved with a simple, one-two-three answer.

For this reason, we do not presume to tell any patient or family members—or any reader of this book—why we think God has allowed their particular trauma to happen to them. We refuse because we don't know! But we have found that those patients and family members who come to a peaceful conviction about an answer often find meaning in one of the four explanations presented in the remainder of this chapter and in the next one. We can affirm these people in these answers, agreeing that these are well-grounded in both Scripture and the experience of many believers. They may be helpful to you as you search for meaning and answers in your own situation.

Answer #1: Cancer Is a Test from God

The first answer that is well-grounded both in Scripture and personal experience is that cancer could be a test sent from God (or allowed by him). This is the answer given in that great treatise on God and suffering, the Book of Job.

Job's afflictions came about as a result of an argument between God and Satan. Satan argued that Job was righteous and faithful to God only because God bribed him.

> "Does Job fear God for nothing?" Satan replied. "Have you [God] not put a hedge around him and his household and everything he has? You have blessed the work of his hands, so that his flocks and herds are spread throughout the land. But stretch out your hand and strike everything he has, and he will surely curse you to your face."[5]

So God agreed to let Satan test Job, if only to prove that there was a man on earth who "fears God and shuns evil."[6]

When Job refused to charge God with wrongdoing after losing his flocks and children, Satan demanded permission to strike Job's body. God consented again. And yet, though Satan expected Job to curse God and Job's wife told him to do so, Job refused. He argued bitterly with God, protesting his innocence, demanding to know why God sent these horrible afflictions, and cursing the day he was born. But Job never cursed God.

Although God never gave Job a direct answer to why these afflictions were sent his way, the reader is told at the very beginning that Job's torments are a test, a way of proving a point to the cosmic powers. If Job had known this, he might have felt honored. After all, God presumably chose him because "there is no one on earth like him"[7]— no one else as God-fearing. God apparently trusted Job to be able to withstand the test of suffering.

The notion that God sends us horrifying pain because he trusts us is unsettling, to say the least. David Watson wrote in exasperation,

> I frankly wish that God did not trust me so much! I would be quite content with less trust on his part and less suffering on mine. It would be a curious way of showing his love to me, and I cannot imagine that I could even think of inflicting such a thing on my children, had I the power to do so.[8]

And yet some people have found a deep sense of peace and meaning in the notion that God has entrusted them with the ordeal of cancer. One such person was Bo Neuhaus, a young boy who wrote the story of the twelfth—and last—year of his life in the moving book, *It's Okay, God, We Can Take It.* This young Texan, who suffered the ravages of liver cancer for more than two years before succumbing to the disease, felt honored to have been given what he considered a test. Two months before his death, he was asked by a family friend if he had ever gotten angry that he'd gotten cancer. "No," Bo replied. "I figured someone had to do it, and I am just sorta proud that God chose me."[9]

The conviction that his suffering was a God-given test gave Bo strength to endure. During one of his chemotherapy sessions, Bo's mother became angry at God because she felt he had taken her beyond her limit. For two nights in a row, Bo had been up all night vomiting, unable to sleep, and his mother had stayed awake to help him. Later, when he heard his mother crying about the ordeal, he told her, "It's not for us to decide how long or how hard God's test is to be—it is only our responsibility to endure it."[10]

Many of us have a hard time accepting this notion of cancer as a test of faithfulness. It seems pointless, for one thing. More disturbing, it seems to assume that God does not know what the outcome will be.

After all, if God knows all things, including the future, why does he need to test us?

C. S. Lewis, the British medievalist and Christian writer who lost his wife to cancer after a brief marriage, speculated in his journal after her death that God may test our faith for our sake, not his. He already knows how we will respond, but we don't, and the experience of testing can teach us a lot about ourselves. Lewis wondered, for example, if part of what God was doing in allowing his wife's death was to show him the flaws in his faith. "[God] always knew that my temple [of faith] was a house of cards. His only way of making me realize the fact was to knock it down."[11]

Answer #2: Cancer Is God's Way of Turning Us to Him

Lewis's reasoning seems contrived to many believers. Yet some who reject his argument nevertheless see in it a grain of truth—that God uses pain to work in people's lives. They see pain, including cancer, as one of God's tools for turning people away from themselves and turning the world toward him. Many can point to patterns in history that they believe illustrate God's use of trouble and trauma to gather people to himself. For example, it was widely reported during the Gulf War of 1991 that churches across the country were filled with more worshipers and seekers than before the war.

Breaking Through Our Self-Sufficiency

Though David Watson could not accept the idea that his cancer was a test, he did believe God had used suffering as a way to break his self-importance and self-sufficiency. Cancer, he wrote, can teach a person—particularly someone who is used to "pulling his own strings"—that he is really not able to control his own life.

Other cancer patients have made the same discovery. When you are being treated for cancer, it quickly becomes apparent that your destiny is in the hands of others—and in the hands of God. Doctors' treatment may enable you to survive; family may have to provide for needs you once took care of yourself. And there are no guarantees. No one can predict the course of your cancer with any certainty, and the question of whether you will even survive is out of your hands. Many cancer patients find this series of realizations pushes them to confront the reality of God for the first time in their lives.

Pain has a way of showing us that something is wrong in life.[12] It forces us to consider other values. With the threat of death looming on the horizon, things that used to seem so important (money, status, house, cars, prestige) suddenly seem trivial. A person who may never have been concerned with religion may be motivated for the first time to seek God.

God's Megaphone

Pain is "God's megaphone to a deaf world," says C. S. Lewis;[13] it magnifies what God says about what is really important in life. And it does this by first shattering the illusion that all is well, then puncturing the myth that what we have is our own and enough for us. It takes out of our hands the things that keep us from receiving what God wants to give.

This can happen to us even if our pain is not physical. Some cancer patients never have physical pain, but the pain of fear and uncertainty can be as great or greater than physical pain. And the friends and relatives of cancer patients may feel as much or more emotional pain than the patients themselves. Cancer can thus become the megaphone through which God calls to a circle of people around the cancer patient, not just the cancer patient.

In his moving spiritual autobiography A Severe Mercy, Sheldon Vanauken chronicles the birth of his faith during and after his wife Davy's terminal illness. Both had started attending church while he studied at Oxford. When they returned to Virginia to teach college English, Sheldon realized that he was no longer the center of Davy's life—that her first love was now for God—and he became jealous of God for Davy's affections.

Then Davy contracted a rare disease and died after a long illness. Looking back, Sheldon realized that her death was in fact a "severe mercy" from God. If she had not died, he believed, his jealousy might have grown to the point that he hated both God and Davy. In her absence, however, he was led to seek, and came to know God on his own. Vanauken writes,

> If my reasoning—my judgment—is correct, then her death in the dearness of our love had these results: It brought me as nothing else could do to know and end my jealousy of God. It saved her faith from assault. It brought me, if Lewis is right [C. S. Lewis had become their friend at Oxford], her far greater help from eternity. And it saved our love from perishing in one of the other ways that love could perish. Would I not rather our love go through death than hate?[14]

Answer #3: Cancer Is God's Way of Making Us Better People

The next answer to the why question is similar to the last one. Once again, the answer focuses on how God uses pain to prepare us for himself.

But while the last reason emphasized the final goal of suffering (bringing us to God), this one looks at what pain does to our inner character.

From God's Image to God's Likeness

Thousands of believers during the past three millennia have testified that this answer made the most sense in their experience of suffering. God seemed to use suffering in their lives to make them better people. As theologians have explained it, God's intent is to perfect our souls. We were created in God's image—that is, we have minds and souls. Now, however, we are called to allow ourselves to be transformed into God's likeness—that is, to move toward spiritual and moral perfection.

God wants us to voluntarily change our actions and hearts to conform to his divine standards. We'll call this voluntary change God's

Plan A. The problem, though, is that we usually don't cooperate. We tend to dislike Plan A because it requires us to change. After all, change often hurts, and it always takes effort. More often than not, our answer is, "No, thanks, God; I'd rather stay the way I am."

When we resist Plan A, God resorts to Plan B. He permits evil and suffering (much of which we bring on ourselves anyway) to come into our lives in order to get us moving toward the goal of spiritual and moral perfection. In other words, God is forced by our own stubbornness and laziness to permit evil and suffering in order to get us to change.* Because we refuse to change ourselves, God gives us a hand. And pain and suffering are our best motivators, our best tutors in this school of character called life.

But Once Again . . . Why?

Now this kind of discussion about God and suffering raises all kinds of questions. Why, for instance, didn't God simply create us good in the first place? Why should we go through all this pain to become good?

Philosophers tell us that if God had created us good, with no chance of being evil, we would not be human beings. This is because part of what it means to be human is to have free will. If God had created us without the freedom to choose evil, we would not have free will, and would therefore be programmed robots rather than human beings.

Without free will, we would miss most of the joy and all of the meaning involved in being human. And we would not fulfill the purpose for which God created us: to live in close relationship with one another and with him.

Another question this talk about God raises is this: Why do we need to become so good in the first place? Why doesn't God just allow us to be morally mediocre? Why torture us with suffering in order to raise us to a standard we don't really care about?

People of faith have answered this question in a similar way for centuries. The answer has to do with our happiness. God knows that we

---

*We are using human terms here to talk about the way God deals with human beings; strictly speaking, if God is all-powerful, he is not forced to do anything.

won't reach the happiness he intends for us as long as we are morally and spiritually mediocre. He knows that moral and spiritual poverty (where most of us live today) in the long run leads only to despair. Suffering hurts, but if we respond to it properly, we can begin to experience a level of happiness that would never have been possible without it. God is too loving to allow us to settle for what will cause us only unhappiness in the long run.

A parent-child analogy has helped many people, especially parents, understand this dynamic a bit more clearly. Parents who truly love their children would rather see those children suffer than remain spoiled and immature. Only a baby-sitter who doesn't really love the children is happy as long as the children do not cry. Naturally, parents would prefer that their children listen to their suggestions and choose maturity. But few children are so compliant. Most don't mature until they have sat through some tough lessons in the school of hard knocks.

Another helpful analogy is that of an artist's work. An artist, as C. S. Lewis once pointed out, will take endless trouble over a masterpiece and inflict endless trouble upon that canvas or marble, with scraping and chipping, as if the work were actually alive and conscious.

And what about a lover? One who loves deeply will be very concerned about how the beloved looks and acts. He will hurt when she hurts, but he'll be willing to suffer with her (rather than alleviating her suffering) if he knows the suffering is necessary for her to become a better person.

Thousands of believers through the centuries have testified after suffering that each is a child of the loving heavenly Father, a work of art on the divine artist's easel, the beloved of the divine lover. We might wish for less pain, but in so doing we are wishing for less love, not more. If we are to let God be God, we must allow him to be repelled by the stains in our character and apply to us the suffering needed to erase those stains.

Three Ways

The Bible has a lot to say about the ways in which suffering makes us better people.

The apostle Peter, for instance, wrote that suffering can deepen and refine faith.[15] David Watson, quoted earlier in this chapter, is an illustration of this. Watson's cancer forced him to reconsider priorities in his life and plunged him deeper into the Bible and the life of God than ever before. In the midst of his battle with cancer, he wrote,

> As I turn to the Bible, I find passages coming alive for me, perhaps more than ever before. . . . I am [now] content to trust myself to a loving God whose control is ultimate and whose wisdom transcends my own feeble understanding.[16]

The apostle James wrote in his Epistle that suffering helps make the believer mature.[17] Bo Neuhaus, the twelve-year-old boy who died of liver cancer, exemplified this kind of maturity forged in pain. His journal gives vivid testimony to the enormous spiritual and emotional growth that cancer helped produce in a young boy. As he struggled against cancer with the weapons of faith, Bo acquired and shared a wisdom far beyond his years.

But the New Testament also declares that suffering produces perseverance and character and thus helps conform us to the image of Christ. And in a particularly surprising passage, the New Testament declares that Jesus himself was perfected through suffering.[18]

A World without Pain?

So from the biblical writers to present-day theologians and philosophers, believers have seen pain as something God uses to make us better people. But perhaps this is still too much for you, particularly if you are philosophically minded. Perhaps you are asking why an all-powerful God could not have produced character in us without this horrible device of pain.

We would respond by challenging you with another question: Is character possible without pain?[19]

Consider the kind of world we would have without pain. Fire would give heat to warm us, but would suddenly lose its heat whenever it was about to cause pain. Water would lose its properties as soon as someone was about to drown. Every time a person was about to suffer pain because of some aspect of the physical environment, a guardian angel would suspend the laws of nature and that person would continue blissfully along. Each time someone was about to be hurt because of a lie or a malicious word, God would intervene to prevent those hurtful words from being spoken.

What kind of human race would result? Certainly not a courageous and wise one, for there would be no risks to brave or dangers to avoid. Instead, human beings would be simple-minded and fragile, never having been toughened by pain or challenged by the threat of failure.

Would true goodness be possible in this world? We don't think so. For how could you have mercy when there are no hurts that need to be forgiven? How can you have courage when there is never any danger? What does honesty mean if telling the truth never has any painful effects?

The examples could go on and on. How can you have determination and perseverance when there are no painful obstacles that must be overcome? How can you have self-sacrifice when no one is ever in need? How can you have compassion when there is no suffering to evoke it? And most important, how can you have altruistic love when there is no cost involved in loving or no lack to be remedied by love?

We believe it would be impossible, then, to develop a capacity to love in a world in which there is no suffering. Goodness would be largely absent in a world where there is no evil.

It's Always a Process

Perhaps you are still skeptical. You are suffering now because you or your loved one has cancer. You don't feel you are becoming a better person. If anything, you're worse: you are cranky, irritable, angry, and frustrated. You don't have your usual love and patience for others because you are so tormented inside.

Don't despair. This process of becoming a better person is exactly that: a process. Most cancer patients and their loved ones don't see character developing in them until long after the crisis originally hits.

Sometimes it takes years. But it does happen—and more often than you might think.

Sure, there are some who go through the ordeal of cancer and are left with only bitterness and rage. Talk of moral and spiritual improvement elicits only a sneer. But there are many more who say they have come away from cancer as better people with bigger hearts and clearer eyes.

Each of us (Bill and Gerry) has had close relatives who have had cancer; some have died, some have survived. Bill has treated cancer patients every day for years. Gerry has known cancer patients and their families both as a pastor and as a religion professor. And both of us have seen more heroes than cynics emerge from this painful experience. In the people we have known, cancer has tended to produce more virtue than vice.

A Biblical Case History

We'll close this chapter with a story from the Bible—the story of a terrible physical problem with which the apostle Paul struggled. Before we begin the story, however, we need to rid ourselves of some false assumptions regarding this leader of the early church.

Many of us have assumed that, since he was so effective in spreading the Christian faith, Paul must have been a charismatic superman. Certainly, we suppose, he must have been a powerful speaker. The evidence we have, however, indicates that he was not a dynamic speaker at all. The Christians at Corinth, for instance, reported that "his speaking amounts to nothing."[20] A Winston Churchill he was not.

We may also be surprised to discover that Paul was probably not tall, strapping, and good looking. One tradition handed down by the early church states that he was short, bald, bowlegged, and homely; his eyebrows are even said to have run together in the middle! A Tom Cruise he was not.

A Thorn in the Flesh

Besides being fairly ordinary in speech and probably ordinary in appearance, Paul suffered from an agonizing physical torment that he called his "thorn in the flesh." What was this thorn in the flesh? Paul never specifies in his letters, and scholars have debated this puzzle for centuries. Some have speculated that he suffered from epilepsy. Other theories have ranged from headaches to depression to leprosy—and even his wife!

What do we know about this thorn in the flesh? We know it came upon him fourteen years before he wrote about it, when he was first preaching in Galatia (a portion of modern Turkey). We know from his letter to the Christians in Galatia that a sickness he contracted there brought him contempt and scorn. He said in that letter that the Galatians then were so kind to him that they would have torn out their eyes and given them to him. Furthermore, he spoke at the end of the letter about the large letters he used as he wrote in his own hand.[21] For these reasons, some scholars believe that he had something wrong with his eyes.

We also know that there was a disease common then in that part of Asia Minor, which intermittently damaged eyesight and also disfigured the face, so that the sufferer looked repulsive. Some scholars have speculated that Paul suffered from this disease, but there is no way to know for sure.

It is clear from the passage in his second letter to the church at Corinth[22] that Paul went through a fair amount of agony over his affliction—a pain that was probably more emotional than physical, caused by humiliation and frustration. Imagine his trying to preach the gospel while noticing that people were distracted by his face and unable to concentrate on his words. This would be particularly aggravating if he were not a powerful speaker in the first place. Perhaps he prayed, "God, this thorn in my flesh is an impediment to the gospel. Surely you want it removed. Just think how much more effective I would be if I were healed! Besides, this is from Satan! Certainly you would not want me to have anything that is of the devil!"

God's Response to Paul

God's response to Paul's first prayer is curious; he said nothing at all. So Paul prayed again. Perhaps he thought he didn't pray hard enough the first time. Again there was no response. Maybe this time Paul felt that he didn't have enough faith. So he prayed a third time. Finally God spoke: "My grace is sufficient for you, for my power is made perfect in weakness."[23]

What did God mean by this? There are a number of implications that can be of help as we seek answers for the question of why God allows cancer.

1. God did not want Paul to be physically healed. Cancer patients need to be aware that the biblical God did not always want to heal; he did not always consider it the best remedy. Christians sometimes assume that physical healing must be God's perfect will for every sick person, but this biblical passage indicates that this is a false assumption.

   When healing doesn't come, some people become bitter toward God because he didn't do what they thought he had promised. But Scripture never promises that God intends physical healing for all. Instead, it affirms that for each person there is "a time to die" and that a person's "days are determined." "All the days ordained for me," wrote the psalmist David, "were written in your book before one of them came to be." Even death, according to the Bible, can be in God's will for a person: "Precious in the sight of the Lord is the death of his saints."[24]

2. God did not want this "messenger of Satan" (Paul's words for the thorn in the flesh) removed! As in the story of Job, God apparently is content sometimes to use the devil's works for God's larger purposes.

3. God wanted Paul to remain weak because only in weakness could Paul experience Christ's grace and power. This can be an important lesson for us when our cancer or a loved one's cancer has brought us face to face with our own helplessness.

What was Paul's response to this message from God regarding his physical torment? He was able to feel gratitude:

Therefore I will boast all the more gladly about my weaknesses, so that Christ's power may rest on me. That is why, for Christ's sake, I delight in weaknesses, in insults, in hardships, in persecutions, in difficulties. For when I am weak, then I am strong.[25]

Paul learned, then, that his sufferings were permitted by God so that he (Paul) could experience new spiritual peace and strength. He was not able to experience this strength as long as he was healthy and strong. For some reason, he had to be weak in order to access this hidden dimension of the spirit. Perhaps your suffering, too, is simply an open door leading to a new experience of grace and power.

Yes, But . . .

On the other hand, you may be thinking that Paul never died from his thorn! Your cancer, or your loved one's cancer, may be life threatening. And you may be asking, What good is this new character if I (or he or she) won't live long enough to experience it?

Believers who have grappled with the question of evil and suffering offer two responses to that question. The first is made by those who hold to the explanation that God produces character through suffering. They say that this new character will make the person better fit to enjoy God in eternity. The person will enjoy more of God because of a greater spiritual depth and may even be able to accomplish more for God in heaven. (These believers argue, on biblical grounds, that the residents of heaven will be up and doing, perhaps even ruling, rather than lying around on clouds and playing harps for eternity.)

But there are many other believers who simply cannot accept any of the explanations offered thus far. They fervently believe in God and may even believe that nothing, even cancer, is outside of God's control. But none of the previous explanations satisfies them completely. Perhaps every attempt to answer why seems to them to carry elements of either sinful pride or silly presumption. Or perhaps they have become convinced that there simply are no answers that we finite humans can comprehend.

We must confess that, although we can see the value of some of the answers we have explored, we must ultimately fall into this last category. That brings us to the next chapter, and the final answer.

11

What to Think When There Are No Answers

Coming to Terms with God's Mystery

Remember Floyd, whose three-year-old son was diagnosed with leukemia? Floyd was horrified by his neighbor John's suggestion that Jimmy's cancer might have been a punishment sent from God. That answer seemed too unfair and inappropriate to be taken seriously. Still searching for answers, Floyd then went to his pastor, who suggested the range of possibilities we presented in the last chapter. Floyd could see the point behind all of these answers, but he still felt completely lost because none of them really seemed to help.

If God was testing him, for instance, Floyd didn't think he was doing very well. He certainly didn't feel honored. Besides, why would a loving God hurt an innocent little boy just to test Floyd?

Neither did Floyd think he was being drawn closer to God because of Jimmy's cancer. After his divorce, before cancer appeared on the scene, he thought he was drawing closer to God. But now the cancer seemed to be creating a distance.

And the idea that his experience might make him a better person left Floyd even further in the dark. Instead of sensing new virtue or stronger character within himself, Floyd could see only a growing anger and bitterness—and confusion. He simply could not sort out the answers to the why question.

Which is why he jerked to attention when a new friend at the hospital, another parent whose child was also being treated for cancer, suggested, "You know, I've thought a lot about this, and I've decided that maybe there just aren't any answers—at least not any we can understand."

When We Don't Know Why

There are many ways to answer the cosmic questions, Why is there suffering? and, more specifically, Why would an all-loving and all-powerful God inflict a three-year-old (or a thirty-three-year old) with cancer?

And for most of us, there comes a time when we must simply shake our heads and say, "I don't understand why." Despite millennia of human experience, despite centuries of scientific exploration, despite the suggested answers of philosophers and poets and researchers and prophets, we all reach a point when we smash our noses flat against the deep mystery at the heart of the universe. We all reach a point when we simply can't know the answers to why.

Is it really surprising that suffering is mysterious? After all, theoretical physicists tell us that the smallest particles of matter are impossible for us to picture. If we make a mental picture to illustrate quantum physics, we move farther away rather than nearer to reality. It should be no surprise, then, that the highest spiritual realities cannot be explained in terms we can understand.

Consider this in another way. If God's intellect is limitless and ours finite, the mystery of evil in the world is just what we might expect. A God of infinite intelligence would probably work in ways that cannot be understood by minds of far less than infinite intelligence. In fact, a universe created by an infinitely intelligent God that was totally comprehensible to finite minds would not make sense.

In a way, mystery may even be beneficial. For think of it—without mystery, there would be far less exercise of truth. It is when suffering seems haphazard and unmerited—incapable of being morally rationalized—that we are more likely to be moved to compassion. If I believe that my neighbor has cancer because God is punishing him for his sins, I will probably have little compassion for him. But if I shake my head in disbelief because he seems so undeserving of such a cruel fate, I will be more inclined to exercise compassion.

The story of Job is a classic illustration of the view that suffering is mysterious. Though at the end of the story God finally gave an answer to Job's long speeches of protest, God never really explained Job's suffering. Instead, God only pointed to his mighty works of creation and reminded Job of his power and greatness.

And Job got the point. After getting this glimpse of God's power, Job threw his face into the dust and said,

> Surely I spoke of things I did not understand,
> things too wonderful for me to know. . . .
> My ears had heard of you
> but now my eyes have seen you.
> Therefore I despise myself
> and repent in dust and ashes.[1]

In the face of God's power and majesty, Job realized that he knew virtually nothing—and that his demand to fathom all the answers to his suffering was both foolish and unreasonable. The lesson for us, as Watson put it, is that we must appreciate our smallness and inability to grasp more than a tiny fraction of total reality. We should not be consumed with why, but simply concentrate on "What are you saying to me? What are you doing in my life? What response do you want me to make?"[2]

We are told from the beginning that Job's suffering was a test of his fidelity. And yet Job himself never saw that bigger picture. He never got a direct answer to his agonized why.

The implication seems to be that mystery will remain part of the human condition. There may be a divine explanation of earthly suffering, but the full explanation is usually not given to us while we tread earthly sod. There will always be some questions we must end up answering, "I just don't know."

Would Knowing Why Really Help?

Some have suggested that, in some cases, understanding why might in fact make matters worse. Joni Eareckson Tada was an athletic seventeen-year-old when a diving accident left her paralyzed from the neck down. During her lengthy hospital stays, her physical and mental suffering was intense. Though a committed Christian, she kept asking why, and the result was only anger and frustration.

A wise friend told her, "You don't have to know why God let you be hurt. The fact is, God knows—and that's all that counts. Just trust him to work things out for good, eventually, if not right away."

"What do you mean?" asked Joni.

"Would you be any happier if you did know why God wants you paralyzed? I doubt it. So don't get worked up trying to find meaning to the accident."[3]

David Watson came to believe during his battle with cancer that persisting with the why question only increased his sense of frustration and perhaps even bitterness. "We only add to our injury and block the way for God's love to reach us."[4]

Bo Neuhaus's mother tells a similar story. Bo regarded his cancer as a kind of test, but even that understanding did not answer all of Bo's questions—and it certainly didn't answer them for Bo's mother. Finally, she gave up trying to figure out why her athletic twelve-year-old son had been stricken with terminal cancer. It seemed impossible to get an answer. But she finally discovered that, emotionally and spiritually, it's easier "to simply trust than to try to figure out God's plan, because one can't find a solution."[5]

Many believers have concluded that what is finally important is not whether we understand why we have cancer but how we respond to that circumstance in our lives.

Watson tells the story of two fathers who came to see him within the space of two months. Each had lost a young child to tragic circumstances. One, a four-year-old, had died of leukemia, while the other, a five-year-old, had drowned in the family's backyard swimming pool.

> One father had been a professing Christian before the disaster but became a bitter and militant atheist as a result; the other had been a professing [secular] humanist but became a committed Christian as a result. They both had roughly the same suffering to contend with, but their reactions were widely different. One had his bitterness to endure as well as his suffering, which in the long run might well have been worse—it was certainly worse for other people; the other found the peace and love of Christ, which transformed his suffering. In all our afflictions, it is not so much our situation that counts but the way in which we react to it. And our reactions can affect, to a remarkable degree, the outcome of our lives.[6]

And that, perhaps, is where we eventually need to leave our struggles with the questions of suffering and evil—and cancer—in the world. There is probably no way we can avoid the whys entirely—not if we're honest with ourselves. And there are many partial answers that can afford us a measure of understanding. But there will always be a point where we must admit that the final answers are beyond us. And it is at that point that we can lay down the burden of pondering why and move on to the question that can really make a difference in our lives— What now?

12

How Do I Cope?

Sources of Spiritual Peace and Strength

How can you cope with the shocking discovery that you have cancer and the ongoing, often painful, process of recovery? You may not be able to answer all your whys, but there is much you can do to ease the pain (physical or emotional) and fear. Among the best is to seek the advice of a good oncologist (cancer doctor) and then to follow it. Many cancers are treatable; if caught in time, they can be cured and life can resume nearly as before. Your doctor will probably recommend a number of strategies to help you deal with the pain and fear. We will touch on a number of them in this chapter but will focus most of our attention on the dimension of life that we believe enhances all the others and may in fact bring the most relief when cancer strikes: the spiritual dimension.

Bill has often noticed the striking difference that a vital faith can make in cancer patients. Patients who have no faith, he has found, are troubled and often panic-stricken. He compares them to a drowning person who cannot swim. Rather than cooperating with would-be rescuers, they pull the rescuers down with them. Relatives, friends, and doctors come to help, but the patients' desperate dependence can make these helpers feel overwhelmed, even suffocated. Because nonbelieving patients fail to see the importance of spiritual wellness and are interested only in physical health, they tend to put unbearable demands and expectations on the shoulders of the people near them. They do this, of course, because for them this life is all there is. Death is the final horror, and they cling to people near them as protection from what they consider to be extinction.

Patients with faith, on the other hand, are also troubled, yet often strong as well. There is fear, and there may be pain, but there is also inner calm. These patients know that if death comes, it is not the end, and this conviction brings a sense of peace. Patients with faith also know that ultimately they cannot depend on human beings alone for recovery, that God is the ultimate source of health. So they do not cling desperately to friends and doctors. Other people come to help and to love, but they often go away strengthened and uplifted by the patients' faith.

Perhaps you are without faith and wonder how to get it. Or maybe you have a little faith but feel a long way from the kind of assurance we just described. How do you break through the anger, fear, and bewilderment in order to feel the comfort? Whether you are trying to determine why God has allowed you to have cancer or are convinced that God doesn't give that kind of knowledge, the biggest task remains: finding God's love and comfort. How do you experience God at the time when you need him the most? This chapter will offer a number of suggestions gleaned from patients who have been there.

Don't Be Afraid to Argue with God

Cancer patients often feel guilty because they find themselves feeling angry at God. They think that such feeling is sin and that any attempt to question God's ways must border on impious blasphemy. Yet some of history's greatest men and women of faith have concluded that arguing with God can be an expression of true faith.

In the Bible's story of Job, for instance, Job spends most of thirty chapters arguing with his friends and with God himself. Job protested that his suffering was unjust because he had been a righteous man. And although God never directly answered Job's accusations, at the end of the biblical story God restored to Job twice what he had before. Before his trials, Job had seven thousand sheep, three thousand camels, five hundred yoke of oxen, and five hundred donkeys. After the trial God gave him fourteen thousand sheep, six thousand camels, a thousand yoke of oxen, and a thousand donkeys.

Now, in the Hebrew law, double restitution was one of the rules for things taken wrongfully.[1] What is the author of Job trying to say? He may have been saying that, although Job was wrong in failing to see the greatness and freedom of God, he was not wrong to accuse God of wrongdoing! Job's faithfulness consisted in not renouncing God even while he argued with him. He may have been self-deceived when he claimed not to have any sin, but he never yielded to his wife's suggestion to curse God. Instead of walking away from God in disgust, he kept searching for God. Rather than giving up, he persisted in his attempts to understand what God was doing. In this sense, he proved his faith by remaining to battle it out with God.

Moses was another great Bible hero who argued with God—and even won some arguments. Once he got God to change his mind about destroying Israel by arguing that God would be breaking a previous promise to multiply the Hebrew nation astronomically. Another time Moses persuaded God to renege on a threat to abandon Israel during its journey through the wilderness. Moses argued that without God's presence, the nation of Israel would lose its distinctiveness in the eyes of the surrounding nations.[2]

Many of us are daunted by the thought of arguing with God. Isn't such arrogance permitted only to the superstars of the faith? Yet the Bible tells us that we should pray like its great heroes[3]—and Moses and Job, like Jacob at the river Jabbok, wrestled with God. If these great people of God wrestled and argued with their Maker, so can we. And just as Jacob finally got a blessing after wrestling with the angel of the Lord all night long, just as Moses found God's grace and love after arguing with God, we too may come to an experience of God's grace and love through faithful argument.

We would go so far as to say that in some cases it is better to dispute with God than to just endorse his policies without question. That is, sometimes we simply must battle it out with God, for by battling we may open ourselves up to an experience of God. If we battle with steadfast purpose and sincerity of heart, we will get an answer, even if God proves us wrong. Job did not get the answer he sought, but by arguing with God he came to an experience of God's glory and power. That experience silenced him, but the silence was a satisfied silence. He no longer needed to have the why question answered.

As Jewish writer Elie Wiesel has put it, "The Jew may love God, or he may fight with God, but he may not ignore God."[4] Arguing with God is a kind of fighting, but even fighting may be an expression of faith. Similarly, a civil rights leader in the 1950s once told his opponents that active hatred was better than indifferent toleration: "Love me or hate me! But don't tolerate me!"

Of course, in arguing with God there is no guarantee that he will "change his mind." Sometimes God says no, as he did to both Moses and Paul. Moses asked to see God's face but was refused; and he was not allowed to go into the Promised Land.[5] Paul asked three times to have his "thorn in the flesh" removed, but God refused, saying that Paul would experience more of Christ's grace by living with his painful ailment.

But even if God says no at the end of the argument, at least a connection has been maintained. The believer has engaged the living God, showing that he or she does not regard God with indifference, but takes him with all seriousness. John Claypool stated this eloquently in a sermon preached just a month after his eight-year-old daughter's death from leukemia: "There is more honest faith in an act of questioning than in the act of silent submission, for implicit in the very asking is the faith that some light can be given."[6]

Don't Be Surprised if God Is Silent

Even as you question and argue with God, however, you should not be surprised if God seems silent during the time you believe you need him most. Although conventional wisdom would indicate that we feel closest to God in times of trouble, the experience of many believers is just the opposite.

Grady had suffered from diabetes since the age of twelve. By the time he reached his midforties, the disease had caused so much damage to his heart, eyes, and kidneys that Grady was forced to quit his job as a computer systems analyst. Before long he had lost 40 percent of his eyesight and had to begin dialysis.

After four years in semiretirement, his life severely constrained by the demands of his treatment, Grady applied for a kidney transplant. But suitable donors were rare, and his age and condition made the odds against his ever getting a kidney almost overwhelming. In spite of the odds, two years later Grady was whisked to a university medical center. A kidney was available.

Grady was elated. A new kidney could restore him to something approaching normal health. He couldn't help imagining the wonderful new freedom he might enjoy. The next six months, however, were a nightmare. As Grady's body slowly rejected the new organ, doctors gave him new, experimental drugs to try to save it. But the cure proved worse than the disease. The drugs brought on painful conditions culminating in strokes and a major heart attack. Grady's body, increasingly unable to sustain all these blows, hovered on the brink of death.

Finally one of the doctors broke the news to Grady: "We're going to have to give up on the transplanted kidney in order to save your life." Although the doctors did not remove the kidney, they gave up their efforts to sustain it. It soon shriveled up, and Grady was back where he started—forced to get dialysis several times a day for the rest of his life. The surgery and other agonies in the hospital had been in vain.

After this setback, Grady reached the lowest point of his life. Although he had had a deep faith for years and had experienced many times when God's love and guidance seemed very real to him, the failure of the transplant threw him into a spiritual tailspin.

Grady knew that God had never promised that the transplant would succeed. But he also knew that donor matches were very difficult to find, and doctors had told him that his age and the advanced state of his diabetes made it unlikely that he would ever be granted one. Having everything fall into place for the transplant had seemed like a miracle—a sure sign of God's blessing.

Grady's hopes had been so high. Now they were cruelly dashed to the ground. The God who had always seemed active and loving in Grady's life seemed suddenly to have abandoned him.

Grady was experiencing what many have experienced during times of great emotional or physical crisis—the silence or seeming absence of God. Even believers who had previously reported many experiences of God's presence and love may have the frightful sense, as C. S. Lewis put it after his wife died, that God "seemed to have his eyes shut, his ears stopped with wax."[7] Prayers go to him, but he doesn't seem to respond. One wonders if he still loves, or ever really did.

Poet Luci Shaw lost her husband Harold to lung cancer after many months of hoping that he would be healed. Luci discovered during the long ordeal that "I find [God] in the light but lose him in the dark." Even after Harold's death, Luci found God's silence to be "deafening."[8]

Lewis went through a similar crisis. But his crisis was curiously ironic because of his earlier writings on God and suffering. *The Problem of Pain*, written in 1944, had argued confidently that pain draws us to God, makes us better people, creates many heroes, and is God's way of training his children. But in his 1961 journal, written during and after his wife's death from cancer, Lewis shared that God had suddenly become a "Cosmic Sadist . . . the spiteful imbecile." Lewis shook his fist at God: "If His ideas of good are so very different from ours, what He calls 'Heaven' might well be what we should call Hell, and vice-versa." At one point during his trauma, Lewis doubted all that he had ever believed about God and Christ; he suspected that his faith may have been just a fragile "house of cards."[9]

Happily, the darkness was eventually lifted for Grady, Shaw, and Lewis, and each learned from his or her experience. After Grady recovered from his surgery, God's love and guiding light came back as before. He says that he learned that God is there, even when he seems to be absent.

Luci Shaw came to realize that God may appear silent, but that he often comes in the guise of other people. Toward the end of her ordeal, she also wondered if perhaps God was teaching her, through the apparent silence, to wait on him:

> For my whole life I have had either a loving father, who wrote home every day when he was away, or a loving husband who made my welfare his concern (as I did his), and who was available for me. Perhaps this availability promoted a kind of dependence that slowed my maturity. If I had a problem or a worry or a decision to make, or a success to share—it was so easy to express it to Harold, and to get his response, that I hardly needed God.
>
> Now I am having to grow up. I have been expecting God to be as instantly available as my husband—to speak to me, to respond in a way that really asked no faith on my part, no waiting, that made no provision for unanswered prayer.[10]

Lewis recovered rather suddenly from his paroxysm of doubt. One morning he woke up and the doubt, along with the heavy burden of grief, had largely vanished. And he learned from the experience that suffering often distorts our perception of God: "You can't see anything properly when your eyes are blurred with tears."

Lewis also concluded that sometimes God does not answer our prayers because our questions are nonsensical. Hence God's silence is not a locked door but . . .

> more like a silent, certainly not uncompassionate, gaze. As though He shook His head not in refusal but waiving the question. Like, "Peace, child; you don't understand."
>
> Can a mortal ask questions which God finds unanswerable? Quite

easily, I should think. All nonsense questions are unanswerable. How many hours are there in a mile? Is yellow square or round? Probably half the questions we ask—half our great theological and metaphysical problems are like that.[11]

Lewis went on to speculate that in heaven we will have our questions answered, but in ways that are totally unexpected:

Not, I think, by showing us subtle reconciliations between all our apparently contradictory notions. The notions will all be knocked from under our feet. We shall see that there never was any problem.[12]

Of course, modern believers are not the only ones who have felt cut off from God during their suffering. Bible heroes sometimes felt the same.

Job's lament throughout his painful experience was that God seemed to be impervious to his suffering, that the heavenly father seemed not to care. Only at the very end of the story, after what could have been months of suffering, did God finally break his silence.

David experienced similar anguish. In Psalm 13 he recorded his exasperation at God's hiddenness:

> How long, O LORD? Will you forget me forever?
> How long will you hide your face from me?
> How long must I wrestle with my thoughts
> and every day have sorrow in my heart?
> How long will my enemy triumph over me?[13]

David went on to write at the end of the psalm that he still trusted in God's unfailing love. He tried to focus on God's past acts of goodness to him. But even these efforts did not totally negate the pain of God's seeming silence.

The prophet Jeremiah had a similar experience. God seemed to have turned against him:

> He has driven me away and made me walk
> in darkness rather than light;
> indeed, he has turned his hand against me
> again and again, all day long. . . .
> He has walled me in so I cannot escape;
> he has weighed me down with chains.
> Even when I call out or cry for help,
> *he shuts out my prayer.*
> He has barred my way with blocks of stone;
> He has made my paths crooked.[14]

Yet Jeremiah was confident that God's silence would end, and that confidence was based on knowledge of God's character:

> Because of the LORD'S great love we are not consumed,
> for his compassions never fail.
> They are new every morning. . . .
> For men are not cast off
> by the LORD forever. . . .
> He does not willingly bring affliction or grief to the
> children of men.[15]

The prophet was convinced that God would restore the joy of his presence in due time.

We can gain important insights from the experiences of Grady, Luci Shaw, C. S. Lewis, David, Job, Jeremiah, and the countless other believers who have found heaven's doors strangely barricaded in times of great suffering. We can realize, for example, that it is not uncommon for believers to feel cut off from God in those times. We can also be assured that the silence—the sense of divine absence—will not last forever, that God will be heard and felt again.

What should you do in the meantime? If you have had meaningful experiences with God in the past, now may be the time to draw on those memories to give you strength. Don't give up on prayer, Bible reading, or church attendance, even though these activities may seem strangely meaningless. (Many people find it helpful to read aloud passages, such as Psalm 13 and Lamentations 3, that cry out to God about his silence.) And don't hesitate to lean on the spiritual strength of others who can pray for you even when your "line" to God seems severed.

Keep hanging in there. Keep talking—to God and to others. Chances are you will find, as so many believers have found before you, that eventually your connection with God will be restored, and you will find he has been there all along.

Remember the Suffering of God

Many Christians who have felt abandoned by God in their suffering have been comforted by remembering that even Jesus felt that way in his time of greatest stress. "My God, my God, why have you forsaken me?" he cried out while hanging naked on the cross. Jesus, too, discovered that in his supreme hour of pain God denied his agonized requests for relief. The Gospel writers portrayed him sweating blood in the Garden of Gethsemane on the night before his brutal scourging and crucifixion. He pleaded three times with God to "take this cup away from me." And no sooner had he finished praying the third time than Judas and a contingent of soldiers appeared. His desperate appeal had been denied! God was going to abandon him to the fullest rigors of an agonizing death.

Meditation on the terrible sufferings of Jesus has comforted and strengthened suffering believers for two thousand years. If Jesus suffered terrible pain and still lives, then two things are true.

1. He understands what I am going through. He knows what it is like to suffer excruciating pain. In a sense, he even dignified our pain by taking it on himself.[16] So even when we are feeling physical or emotional pain, we should never feel alone. Jesus knows what the pain is like, and he suffers it with us.

2. There is hope that just as he received new life through his suffering, so will I. When suffering the side effects of chemotherapy,

twelve-year-old Bo Neuhaus (whose story is told in chapter 10) found that knowing Jesus' sufferings were "harder than this . . . made it more bearable for me."[17] Joni Eareckson Tada, who was paralyzed from the neck down after a diving accident, was strengthened at a critical time when she realized that Jesus had also endured great pain.[18]

Believers can derive great comfort from the conviction that God suffers with them in their suffering. There is ample biblical support for this belief. Isaiah wrote of God's relationship to his people: "In all their distress he too was distressed."[19] Jeremiah also portrayed God as being deeply affected by the discipline of his children:

> Is not Ephraim [one of the tribes of Israel]
>> my dear son,
> the child in whom I delight?
> Though I often speak against him,
> I still remember him.
> Therefore my heart yearns for him;
> I have great compassion for him.[20]

Hosea went on to picture God as suffering when his people were unfaithful:

> How can I give you up, Ephraim?
> How can I hand you over, Israel? . . .
> My heart is changed within me;
> all my compassion is aroused.[21]

And finally, when Lazarus's sisters were grieving his death, Jesus responded with genuine and spontaneous compassion. We are told that "Jesus wept."[22]

But it is Jesus' crucifixion that shows above all else the suffering heart of God. The Bible says that God was in Christ reconciling the world to himself and that Jesus was God—the Word—made flesh.[23] If

Jesus was God in human form, God himself experienced the act of supreme human suffering—hanging naked on the cross, with gnats and flies crawling over his wounds and soldiers mocking and spitting—for the sake of drawing us to him.

If the cross was where God chose to reveal himself most clearly, to perform his supreme saving act in human history, then we have a God who suffers. If God chose to reveal himself in a man who was "acquainted with grief,"[24] then we have a God who suffers. In fact, suffering appears at the very heart of who and what God is.

William Temple once described it this way:

> "There cannot be a God of love," men say, "because if there was, and he looked upon the world, his heart would break." The Church points to the Cross and says, "It did break." "It is God who made the world," men say. "It is he who should bear the load." The Church points to the Cross and says, "He did bear it."[25]

If this is true—if God in Christ suffered on the cross—then we cannot so readily accuse God of injustice when he allows us or our loved ones to be afflicted with pain.

Dorothy Sayers wrote:

> For whatever reason God chose to make man as he is—limited and suffering and subject to sorrows and death—He had the honesty and courage to take His own medicine. Whatever game He is playing with His creation, He has kept His own rules and played fair. He can exact nothing from man that He has not exacted from Himself. He has himself gone through the whole of human experience, from the trivial irritations of family life and the cramping restrictions of hard work and lack of money to the worst horrors of pain and humiliation, defeat, despair and death. When He was a man, He played the man. He was born in poverty and died in disgrace and thought it well worthwhile.[26]

Suffering cancer patients, then, can know that God hurts with them when they hurt. The God who winced when he had to discipline his people and who cried out in pain when nails were driven through his wrists and ankles shares our pain and enters into our sorrows with his compassionate love.

As Lewis put it, we can know that, like a schoolteacher teaching a child how to print, God is holding our hand as we try to trace the difficult letters. Because we are following the example of a suffering God, our script need only be a copy, not an original. He can help us endure our pain because he suffered before us and still suffers with us.

Focus on God and Life with Him

Suffering believers have found not only that God suffers with them but also that he changes their perspective on life. Many eventually come to the realization that this earthly life is not what is finally most important, and this realization has boosted their spirits.

In a letter to his classmates one month before his death, twelve-year-old Bo Neuhaus wrote:

> Although physically I am not doing too well, my spirit and faith are great. I know that God is doing good things even though it is hard to understand sometimes. I have learned that the body is not what's important—what is important is your spirit and faith in God, and if you can keep your spirit and faith way up, you know that everything is going to be okay.[27]

Mario is a sixty-year-old man in my (Gerry's) church who came to a living faith only two years before he contracted cancer. His particular form of cancer was deadly; his doctors had told him that the average life expectancy for a man in his condition was less than a year. In the face of this death sentence, members of the church were astounded by Mario's cheerfulness and radiance. But he told a weekly Bible study group a story that helped explain his good cheer in the midst of dark uncertainty.

"One night several weeks ago," he told his friends, "I was lying in the hospital bed getting a chemo treatment. I was hooked up to so many tubes that I could hardly move. It was about one o'clock in the morning. As I was lying there, unable to sleep because of the irritation and discomfort of all these tubes, God touched me with his love and his peace. I can't describe it, but I can tell you it was fantastic. All I can say is that, after that experience, what have I got to complain about?"

When Mario's friends asked if they could pray for him, he waved them off, telling them they should pray for people with greater needs. He wasn't rejecting their love and concern but simply expressing his sense of peace. He had experienced God so wonderfully that he just wanted others to have that same experience.

Thinking about heaven has also helped many to transcend their daily sufferings. Now, the hope of heaven has been used by some to manipulate people and avoid responsibility—to perpetuate the status quo and reinforce the control of the powerful. Many religious people and groups in the history of Christianity have deserved censure for telling the poor and oppressed to be content with their lot because heaven awaited them—when both the wealthy religious and the poor themselves could have done much to improve their earthly plight.

But cancer patients are in a different situation. Focusing on what awaits them after death—whether the cancer is cured or not—does not usually mean that they are neglecting earthly remedies. In fact, it is often the uncertainty of earthly remedies that leads them to think about heaven. And cancer patients often find that considering heaven makes earth's sufferings more bearable. Death becomes less frightening, and the pain is somehow more easily endured.

Bo Neuhaus, for example, was strengthened throughout his bout with cancer by thinking about heaven. Fairly early in his sickness, he wrote in his journal, "If I die it would be okay; I would be the lucky one in heaven with God and Jesus and it would be a perfect life for me." Then, just two months before his death, Bo told friends that he was not afraid because "I knew I would be in a better life with God and Jesus, and it would be paradise."[28]

These words have a slightly syrupy quality that can make them seem to be artificial platitudes coming from a naive child. But this child had already gone through hell; he had earned his right to be heard. And his insights about the meaning of life after death are the same ones that have brought comfort to many cancer patients.

Listen for God Speaking through Others

Luci Shaw found that God often came to her in the disguise of other people. This is the experience of many who have gone through the ordeal of cancer. Sometimes we may think that God has deserted us when he may in fact be caring for us through friends, technicians, nurses, or doctors. He may be speaking to us through loved ones who give us a word of encouragement or comfort—or even a cry that tells us that someone is suffering with us.

Richard Wurmbrand heard from God that way during a particularly excruciating time of his life. Wurmbrand is a Romanian pastor who spent fourteen years in Communist prisons, where he was repeatedly tortured for his faith in Christ. He remembers, "They broke four vertebrae in my back and many other bones. They carved me in a dozen places. They burned me and cut eighteen holes in my body." But even in the midst of that torture, Wurmbrand heard God speaking through the anguished voice of a fellow prisoner. David Watson tells the story:

> For three years [Wurmbrand] was in solitary confinement thirty feet below ground level, during which time the only persons he saw were his torturers. In despair he asked God to speak to him, to say something to him. At that moment he heard a terrible piercing cry. It was from another victim who was being tortured. But Wurmbrand heard it as a cry from God's heart.[29]

Here, once again, we see the notion of God suffering in our suffering. But we also see Wurmbrand's sense that God came to him—spoke to him—through other human beings.

Try to Look Outside Yourself

Psychiatrists and counselors have found that if they can get patients to see themselves as helpers and givers instead of always receivers, healing may be hastened. (The healing may not be of the physical, but it will certainly be of the emotional.)

Some cancer patients tend to wallow in self-pity; they become self-obsessed, relating everything they experience to their sickness and their needs. Their physical problem therefore becomes an emotional burden that others must painfully bear, and their obsessive focus on their own pain makes the pain seem even more acute. But if these patients can begin to focus on others' needs, their own pain can be blunted—and their relationships will certainly improve.

Mario discovered that was true. Despite his pain and discomfort, he scurried around church trying to do what he could to help others. Joni Eareckson Tada has discovered the same reality. Today she travels around the country, talking about her pain in an effort to help relieve others of theirs. Both these people have experienced the joy of helping others—which certainly does not eliminate their own pain, but which can make the pain more bearable.

Becoming involved in projects outside oneself is another good therapy—as Brian Sternberg discovered. In 1963, track magazines ranked Sternberg as the world's best pole vaulter. That same year, he lost control during a vault and landed on his head. He has been paralyzed from the neck down ever since and lives in constant pain. Although questions still haunt him, he tries to get his mind off the physical and emotional pain by devoting energy to his hobby—amateur radio. When he is talking with people all over the world, developing friendships and helping strangers in need, Brian's pain does not go away, but it does become a little bit easier to endure.[30]

Accept Your Emotions

Both tears and laughter are gifts of God—and you need both to make it through the trial of cancer.

Bo Neuhaus and his mother felt much better after they cried together at the end of a bad day; the tears seemed to lift the burden. David Watson and other cancer patients have had similar experiences. They have learned that a good cry is sometimes the best prescription for intense fear and grief; it can release the heavy emotional burden of the stressful situation. Trying to "keep a stiff upper lip" or "be strong" can get in the way of experiencing a needed emotional release.

Humor can also be therapeutic—and not only in the emotional sense. Norman Cousins's "humor therapy," which helped him recover from what was thought to be an incurable disease, is now famous. He recovered after a planned "humor regimen" of watching taped comedy shows and reading funny stories for hours each day in his hospital bed.

Physiologists tell us that laughter releases endorphins, those magical proteins that enhance the healthy functioning of cells and can give us a feeling of euphoria. (They are the source of what is called the runner's high.) So our modern understanding of the body supports what the biblical writer told us thousands of years ago: "A cheerful heart is good medicine."[31]

For Those Who Want to Help

Before wrapping up this chapter, we want to add a word for those caring for a cancer patient—or those who are supporting the loved ones of a cancer patient. Some people will inevitably try to help the patient or his or her family by explaining how everything "will all work out for the good." They may even be so bold as to suggest that God is using the experience to correct some of the patient's faults. The most reckless and insensitive may proclaim that God is punishing the patient's sins.

But the experience of those suffering indicates that even the best-intentioned word of explanation or biblical encouragement—such as "God had this all planned; there's really nothing to worry about"—will usually fail to comfort and may even do harm. As we have seen, there are no final and certain answers for the why question—at least, none that we finite humans can know. And answers to why are not really what the cancer patient usually needs to hear, anyway.

David Watson remembers that when he was battling cancer, he needed to be reminded of God's love, not his disciplinary designs. He needed not theology but sympathy, not condemnation but affirmation, not cold moralizing but warm compassion.

C. S. Lewis discovered the same reality. He wrote, "When pain is to be borne, a little courage helps more than much knowledge, a little human sympathy more than much courage, and the least tincture of the love of God more than all."[32]

And philosopher Nicholas Wolterstorff, who lost a twenty-five-year-old son in a climbing accident, adds that people who are facing death don't need to hear that death is ultimately not that bad. Instead, they need to hear that we are with them in their desperation. Instead of explanations, they need our compassion, to have us come close and sit beside them on the mourning bench.[33]

Job's comforters have been criticized for centuries because of their pretentious and insensitive attempts to explain to Job why he was suffering. Yet if we would listen to sufferers like Watson and Wolterstorff, we might learn from the example of Job's friends in their first response to the news of Job's tragedies: "They sat on the ground with him for seven days and seven nights. No one said a word to him, because they saw how great his suffering was."[34] Often those who are suffering because of cancer would appreciate a similar response of quiet presence—but no advice—from us.

Another important thing to know for those who want to help cancer victims and their families is that treatment for cancer can be a long, drawn-out affair. It's easy to fall into the trap of showering attention on a friend during the first few weeks after the diagnosis but gradually drifting away as the course of the disease wears on. Listen to the cry of a woman who wrote Ann Landers:

Dear Ann Landers

I'm another one who never thought I would write to you, but a letter in your column struck a chord in my heart. I'm referring to the woman whose husband is unemployed and whose friends have forgotten them. So much of what she said can be applied to us.

My beloved husband, who is only 46, is terminally ill. He has been battling cancer for almost a year and unless we have a miracle, he won't live much longer. I'd like to use your column to speak to our friends and family members who have disappeared into the woodwork.

"Dear Friends and Family: Where are you? Do you know how lonely we are? You were all there in the beginning when the shock was so great—and you gave us strength to get through it. You didn't know what to say, but you came anyway and just sat with us and cried with us and let us know you cared.

"That was almost a year ago. Where have you been since? Do you know how we long to hear the phone ring, to see a car in the driveway or a card in the mail? You don't have to stay long. In fact, it's probably best if you don't. But right now we feel as if we've been abandoned.

"We don't have the plague. Cancer is not contagious and our emotional needs are almost as great as my husband's physical needs. The thing is, I know you'll be there at his funeral to say how sorry you are and offer to help. And then you'll disappear again. And when that happens, you'll wish that you'd called more or tried to visit more often, but it will be too late."

—Hurting in Suburbia[35]

If we want to be sensitive to the needs of our friends and relatives who have cancer, we should keep on visiting and helping over the long term, not just when the news first breaks. When we visit them, we will hug them and cry with them, empathize and pray with them. We will listen to them and reaffirm God's and our own love for them. That love should include physical touch—cancer patients need touching as much as healthy persons do. Without it, they can feel like pariahs or lepers.

Sometimes relatives and friends stay away from cancer patients because they don't know what to say. Perhaps this is why the woman's friends and family stopped coming to visit. But as the woman's letter poignantly demonstrates, the silence of friends and family can be the greatest pain of all. And as Job and his friends have taught us, knowing what to say is of secondary importance to just being there.

13

Dare I
Hope for Healing?

---

*A Balanced Approach to the
Possibility of Getting Well*

W e hope this book is showing you that a diagnosis of cancer need
not be a death sentence. If detected early enough and treated
properly, many cancers can be arrested and even cured. And even
some of the most deadly and far-advanced cancers have surrendered
to the combined attack of medicine and prayer. This chapter tells the
stories of three people who believe that without God's power, they and
their doctors would have been defeated by cancer. Toward the end of
the chapter we explain how you can pray for healing.

Does God Heal Today?—Two Extreme Opinions

The good news is that God can heal cancer and sometimes does. But
before we tell you the stories of people who have been healed by God
of their cancer, we need to deal with two extreme—and, we believe,
false—positions on this question of healing. You may be familiar with
them both.

One Extreme: God Always Wants to Heal

The first extreme position on divine healing is that it is always God's will that we be healed. As we have seen, proponents of this view claim that only our unbelief or sin keeps God from healing us when we are sick. This teaching has filled many with guilt and a sense of condemnation. If they pray for healing but remain ill, they are left with a sense of inner shame or frustration. They have searched their hearts for sin, repented of what they found, but still remain unhealed. So they are tormented with questions:

- Have I committed an unforgivable sin?

- Do I have an unbelieving heart?

- Is God angry with me because I have not been able to muster enough faith for healing?

These and many other questions can torture people who subscribe to this teaching. In some cases, the overwhelming guilt and shame that result have led to deep psychological problems.

People who are agonizing over seemingly unanswered prayers for healing need to be reassured that some of the greatest Bible figures also had experience with such prayers. After the baby born to Bathsheba and David fell sick, for instance, David pleaded with God for its life. He fasted for days and spent his nights lying on the ground. On the seventh day, however, the baby died.[1]

And although Jesus healed many people during his earthly ministry, it apparently was not his will or intention to heal everyone. His healing was sometimes selective. The pool of Bethesda, for instance, was the first-century equivalent of a hospital; dozens of sick people crowded around it in hope of healing. As far as we know, however, Jesus healed only one man out of that suffering crowd.[2]

The apostle Paul also had his share of experience with seemingly unanswered prayers for healing. At one point, for instance, as Paul relates in his letter to the church at Philippi, his friend Epaphroditus became sick. Only after what seemed to be a protracted illness did

Epaphroditus escape death. No doubt Paul prayed for his friend's healing, as he had prayed successfully for others. This time, however, the
prayers had no immediate effect. In fact, Epaphroditus almost died.
Paul must have wondered whether his prayers would go unanswered.[3]

Then, in Paul's second letter to Timothy, he wrote, "I left Trophimus
sick in Miletus."[4] Trophimus was Paul's traveling companion on his
third missionary journey.[5] Again, we can suppose that Paul probably
prayed for Trophimus to be healed, but his prayer for healing was not
answered—at least not in time for Trophimus to travel.

And of course Paul's fervent prayers for the physical healing of his
"thorn in the flesh" were not answered—or were answered with a no.
All of these experiences of the great apostle leave us with a question:
Were Paul's prayers for healing unanswered because of Paul's unbelief
or sin? Or were they indications that God does not always want to heal
us physically?

Paul's first letter to Timothy shows that Paul sometimes chose not
to pray for healing in the face of illness. Timothy had stomach problems, and Paul recommended not prayer but medicine: "Stop drinking only water," he urged his young disciple, "and use a little wine
[thought to have medicinal value in the first century] because of your
stomach and your frequent illnesses."[6] Did Paul pray for Timothy's
healing before advising medical remedies? We don't know, of course;
all we know is that in this case Paul seemed not to believe that God
wanted to heal Timothy through prayer alone.

These events in the lives of biblical people make it clear that, even
in times of miracles, not everybody who prayed for healing was healed.
They also imply that it is not God's will to heal everyone of every illness. As Jesus was selective at the pool of Bethesda, God seems to be
selective in whose prayers for healing are granted.

Why wouldn't God want to heal? We looked at many possible
answers to this question in chapter 10. One that the Hebrew Scriptures
(for Christians, the Old Testament) makes clear, and that bears repeating when considering some cancers, is that each person has an
appointed time to die. In addition, the position that God always wants
to heal is theologically suspect. The Christian tradition has always

affirmed that our bodies will not be redeemed until the kingdom of God is fully realized, which will come only after the return of Christ, or at least after our own deaths. The Bible teaches that the fullness of resurrection life is still to come. To expect healing after every illness is to expect resurrection prematurely.

The early church taught that creation is still in "bondage to decay." Hence full liberation won't come until the final state of perfected glory after the end of the world. Only then will "the perishable . . . clothe itself with the imperishable, and the mortal with immortality."[7]

Sometimes we forget that death can bring a kind of healing. We cling to physical healing and physical life as if they were our highest goods. But Paul recognized that life on this earth, even after physical healing, is only a prelude to a better kind of life: "We are confident, I say, and would prefer to be away from the body and at home with the Lord."[8]

One final word on miracles is needed at this point. If God does grant the miracle of physical healing, he may do this in ways that we don't notice. In June 1991, for instance, a minister friend of ours named Paul was sick with an infectious disease for three weeks and then recovered. No one really thought a miracle had happened; Paul just got well. But just one month later, another adult male about Paul's age was treated in the same hospital for the same disease. This second man went into shock, suffered brain damage, and died forty-eight hours later.

What made the difference? Paul was admitted to the hospital at a slightly earlier stage of the sickness. But how do you explain that? Was that an accident? Or was it a blessing of providence—that is, was it perhaps God's hand that moved Paul to make an appointment before the other man did? If that is what happened, can't we call his healing a miracle—if by miracle we mean God's intervention to save a person from an otherwise fatal disease?

Bill often sees breast cancers discovered at very early stages through mammography. Because of early detection, these cancers are often cured. Why can't we think of God's healing through early detection as well as through other methods?

Too often we make the mistake of thinking that God is involved only when medicine has failed. But, as we shall see later in this chapter, we believe God works through medicine and doctors as well. Perhaps he should be recognized as the One who helps us discover tumors at stages when they are curable. In our minds, that's a miracle as great as any.

The Other Extreme: God Never Heals

The other extreme position on this question of God and healing is that miracles never occur today. Some support this position by appealing to the laws of nature. God, they argue, created the world to operate by the laws of nature. He does not intervene to violate those laws but allows everything in the physical world to proceed in accordance with them. Miracles are not possible, therefore, because they involve suspension of the laws of nature, and God has already committed himself not to suspend those laws.

There are a number of problems with this position, however.

A Scientific Problem

The first problem with the position that God never intervenes in the laws of nature is that it is scientifically outdated! To talk of laws of nature as universal and fixed was typical of Newtonian science from the eighteenth to the early twentieth centuries. Today's physicists, however, regard laws of nature as statistical. That is, they describe what generally occurs; they are not live forces in the universe that cause or keep anything from happening. According to current scientific thinking, therefore, the laws of nature should not be considered a barrier to the occurrence of miracles. In fact, the eminent German physicist Werner Schaafs concludes that "even the physicist must officially concede the possibility of intervention by God."[9]

Using this perspective, a theologian would say that the laws of nature describe how God ordinarily works in the world: God constantly intervenes in nature, but he normally does this in patterns that are referred to as laws of nature. There is no reason why God cannot occasionally step out of his usual pattern of working. The occasional variation in God's working is what is called a miracle.

A Logical Problem

Another problem with the position that God never violates the laws of nature by performing miracles is that it is based on an unproven or a priori assumption. To subscribe to this position, we must assume there are no miracles before we have evidence to support such an assumption. For how can we know for sure that the thousands of people throughout history who have claimed to have experienced a miracle were deceived or lying? There is no way that we can prove or disprove most of their claims. So for us to say that miracles do not occur is to assume, without evidence, that all those claims are spurious. As C. S. Lewis pointed out, this is circular reasoning:

> Unfortunately, we know the experience against [miracles] to be uniform only if we know that all reports of them are false. And we can know all the reports to be false only if we know already that miracles have never occurred. In fact, we are arguing in a circle.[10]

Biblical Problems

A third problem with the position that God does not violate the laws of nature in order to heal people is biblical in nature. The simple fact is that the Bible is full of miracles, and there is no indication that different laws of nature were operating in those days.

Most of us know that the New Testament portrays Jesus healing fevers, leprosy, paralysis, withered hands, blindness, deafness, and hemorrhages. He cast out evil spirits and even raised the dead. Even though he did not heal everyone, healing did comprise a considerable portion of his earthly ministry. In fact, of 1,257 narrative verses on Jesus' ministry in the New Testament, 484 (38.5 percent) describe healing or deliverance from evil spirits. And healing did not stop with Jesus' death and resurrection. After he ascended into heaven, the leaders of the early church continued similar ministries of healing—healing the sick and raising the dead in his name.[11]

Some Christians accept the historicity of the miracles of the early church but believe that miracles stopped after the apostolic era. Miracles were necessary then, they argue, to validate the mission of Jesus and his apostles. Now that the world has seen through those miracles that Christ was sent by God, miracles are no longer needed.

Many healings in the New Testament, however, were performed by Jesus out of compassion, not to validate his ministry. Matthew wrote for instance, that Jesus once saw a large crowd, "had compassion on them and healed their sick."[12] Another time, when Jesus was in Jericho, he heard two blind men shouting over and over again for him to come over to them and "have mercy on us." Matthew recounts that "Jesus had compassion on them and touched their eyes. Immediately they received their sight and followed him."[13] According to the Gospel writers, the purpose of these and similar miracles was not to prove anything about Jesus but simply to care for people and show love for them.

There is no indication that the New Testament authors believed healing miracles would cease after the death of the apostles. Quite the contrary is true, in fact. According to John, Jesus told his followers that they would do even greater miracles than he had done: "Anyone who has faith in me will do what I have been doing. He will do even greater things than these, because I am going to the Father."[14]

In one of the last verses of Mark's Gospel, Jesus predicts that his followers "will place their hands on sick people, and they will get well."[15] This verse was probably not a part of the original Gospel, but it nevertheless indicates the faith of the early church that healings would continue.

The apostle James is even more specific in his Epistle. He directs the church, "Is any one of you sick? He should call the elders of the church to pray over him and anoint him with oil in the name of the Lord. And the prayer offered in faith will make the sick person well; the Lord will raise him up."[16] James made no indication at all that this advice was to become null and void once the apostolic era was over.

We have considerable historic evidence that healings did continue past the early days of the church. For example, Irenaeus (circa 130–202) was a second-century bishop in France who wrote that some "still heal the sick by laying their hands upon them, and they are made whole. Yea, moreover, as I have said, the dead even have been raised up and remained among us for many years."[17]

Augustine (354–430), Christianity's greatest theologian during its first millennium, believed during his early career that miracles had ceased after the death of the apostles. But in his *Retractions*, written three years before his death, he wrote that he had changed his mind after seeing seventy miracles attested in his own diocese in just two years' time. And his great work, *The City of God*, tells of a woman who was healed of breast cancer:

In the same city of Carthage lived Innocentia, a very devout woman of the highest rank in the state. She had cancer in one of her breasts, a disease which, as physicians say, is incurable. Ordinarily, therefore, they either amputate, and so separate from the body the member on which the disease has seized, or, that the patient's life might be prolonged a little, though death is inevitable even if somewhat delayed, they abandon all remedies, following, as they say, the advice of Hippocrates. This lady we speak of had been advised to by a skillful physician, who was intimate with her family; and she betook herself alone to God by prayer.

On the approach of Easter, she was instructed in a dream to wait for the first woman who came out from the baptistery after being baptized, and to ask her to make the sign of Christ upon her sore. She did so, and was immediately cured. The physician who had advised her to apply no remedy if she wished to live a little longer, when he had examined her after this, and found that she who, on his former examination, was afflicted with that disease was now perfectly cured, eagerly asked her what remedy she had used, anxious, as we may well believe, to discover the drug which should defeat the decision of Hippocrates. But when she told him what had happened, he is said to have replied, with religious politeness, though with a contemptuous tone, and an expression which made her fear he would utter some blasphemy against Christ, "I thought you would help me make some great discovery." She, shuddering at his indifference, quickly replied, "What great thing was it for Christ to heal a cancer, who raised one who had been four days dead?"[18]

Reports of physical healing are found in virtually every century since the apostles. Many of these may be counterfeit, of course, but it is still significant to note that there is no sudden decline of reports after the end of the New Testament era. The twentieth century, moreover, has witnessed a veritable explosion of healing claims. This huge increase of reports may be due at least in part to better access to media coverage. But still, if we believe that miracles occurred in the New Testament era, it is difficult to discount the possibility that miracles have occurred since that time.

Theological Problems

Finally, there are theological problems with the view that God never interferes with the ordinary workings of nature. This view keeps God "out there," beyond the experience of everyday reality. Such a God seems distant and somewhat impersonal—quite different from the living and personal God of the Bible and traditional Christian faith. Former Catholic priest Francis MacNutt* has seen hundreds of people healed through his ministry. At one time he, too, was skeptical of the claim that God contravenes nature's laws. But experience has taught him, he says, both that God still heals today and that healing shows God's compassion as little else does:

As a Harvard graduate with a Ph.D. in theology I am as aware as anyone of problems of credulity and of a prevailing theological climate

---

*You will notice that we refer several times in this chapter to MacNutt's ministry and books. We do so because MacNutt's books are the best that we have seen on the subject and the reports of healings that took place through his ministry seem more convincing than others.

which questions whether God "intervenes" or "interferes" in the universe. But my own experience leads me to the conclusion that healing is the most convincing demonstration to most people that God is with us—that he is not "out there" beyond the reach of human compassion. . . .

My own experience has been that a person who has known God's healing love and power senses the presence of God within himself, the immanent God, the God who works in and through his creation. Far from imagining God as distant, I sense him as more present than ever before. He has many ways of acting in our lives. To limit his power by saying that he acts only through nature, does indeed make him seem distant and impersonal. In effect, to insist that God does not heal puts him "out there," makes him an impersonal force, even less involved than any compassionate human being.[19]

What about the Fakes?

After the TV preachers' sex and money scandals of the 1980s, many of us are loathe to consider the possibility of healing today. Their antics and deceptions may ring in our ears when we consider the possibility of healing. But for us to dismiss the possibility of healing because some practitioners have been discredited is to make the common mistake of generalizing about a practice because of the notorious abusers of that practice.

It is widely known, for instance, that some teachers teach with little knowledge and bad motives. And yet we all know that we cannot conclude from that fact that the teaching profession is intrinsically bad. A medical charlatan using a good drug in the wrong way may kill a patient. But that does not mean that the same drug when used properly by a competent physician will not cure disease. And the practice of healing in God's name has been similarly abused. Yet we cannot conclude from that fact alone that it is not possible.

Can Healing Be Psychosomatic?

It is possible, of course, that many healings may be psychosomatic (a result of one's emotional state). Medical research has shown strong correlations between the attitudes of our minds and the conditions of our bodies. But does this mean that every healing can be reduced to emotional fallout?

In our experience, too many healing stories fail to fit a discernible pattern that links an emotional condition with either sickness or health. For every case that fits such a pattern, there is another one that doesn't.

Thus the assumed psychosomatic origin of every claimed healing at this point remains far short of proof. And for believers, there always remains the possibility of supernatural intervention. If at least some of the healings described in the Bible actually happened, and if there is no good reason why similar events could not occur today, then we must keep our minds open to the possibility that God could heal again today.

Our Answer: God Heals Through Medicine and Prayer

Our position differs from the two extremes we have just discussed. We believe that, although God is always loving, God does not always choose to heal us physically. At the same time, we think it would be wrong for a cancer patient to arbitrarily rule out the possibility of divine healing. For we have seen clear evidence that God sometimes works through the combination of medicine and prayer to cure cancer that seems nearly hopeless. We will present some of that evidence in the stories that follow.

Now, evidence is not the same thing as indisputable proof. In each of the stories, chemotherapy was used, and it is possible that the chemotherapy alone is what brought about each healing. Yet the circumstances of each healing, when weighed against the normal odds of recovery, are extraordinary. They are miraculous if by *miraculous* we mean "an otherwise almost inexplicable healing that occurs after prayer to God."[20]

The conjunction of prayer and medicine in these healings demands comment, however. We know of no lasting remission from otherwise hopeless cancers gained from prayer alone—without the use of any medical treatment—that have occurred in recent years.

(Some people undoubtedly claim such healings, but we have not found documentation for any of these.) There are reports of such cases in centuries past, such as the one in Augustine's diocese quoted above, but in all the cases we know of, healing came through both medicine and prayer.

This union of faith and medicine has a long tradition in the Judeo-Christian tradition. For more than two thousand years, both the physician and medicine have been seen as instruments of God's healing. As Ben Sira wrote in the book of Ecclesiasticus (circa 200 B.C.E.):

> Treat the doctor with the honor that is his due,
>> in consideration of his services; for he too has
>> been created by the Lord.
> Healing itself comes from the Most High,
>> like a gift received from a king.
> The doctor's learning keeps his head high,
>> and the great regard him with awe.
> The Lord has brought medicinal herbs from the ground,
>> and no one sensible will despise them.
> Did not a piece of wood once sweeten the water,
>> thus giving proof of its power?
> He has also given some people the knowledge,
>> so that they may draw credit from his mighty works.
> He uses these for healing and relieving pain;
>> the druggist makes up a mixture from them.
> Thus, there is no end to his activities; thanks to him,
>> well-being exists throughout the world.
> My child, when you are ill, do not rebel,
>> but pray to the Lord and he will heal you.
> Renounce your faults, keep your hands unsoiled,
>> and cleanse your heart from all sin.
> Offer incense and a memorial of fine flour,
>> make as rich an offering as you can afford.
> Then let the doctor take over—the Lord created him too—
> and do not let him leave you, for you need him.

There are times when good health depends on doctors,
>   for they, in turn, will pray the Lord to grant them the
grace to relieve and to heal, and so prolong your life.
Whoever sins in the eyes of his Maker, let such a one
>   come under the care of the doctor![21]

In the New Testament, as we have seen, we have the example of Paul recommending a medicinal treatment to Timothy for his stomach ailments. Those who condemn the use of medicine as a failure to trust in God are therefore departing from centuries of counsel in both Judaism and Christianity.

In the stories that follow we can see a similar pattern. All these people used medicine, doctors, and modern technology. All also trusted in God and received abundant prayer. Each case featured extraordinary results that are difficult to explain as the effects of medicine alone.* Nor can the similarity of pattern and results be explained by the age or situation of the three patients; one was a four-year-old girl, another a young man of about twenty years, and the third was a forty-eight-year-old mother of seven.

Roell's Story

Roell's story is an abridged version of an article by Robert J. Byrne in the St. Louis Review and reprinted in Francis MacNutt's book, *The Power to Heal*.[22]

They do not claim that a miracle has occurred. However, the parents of four-year-old Roell Ann Schmidt of St. Roch Parish here firmly believe that God cured their daughter of cancer.

Moreover, they believe that God acted in response to very specific prayers for healing, as offered weekly by Catholics who themselves firmly believe in the power of prayer to heal.

---

*In the 1990s these types of tumors are cured more often, though still infrequently. The fact that these people were healed in the 1970s and 1980s, when treatment methods were less developed, is truly remarkable.

Their belief is buttressed by the physicians and surgeons from St. Louis Children's Hospital who decline to take credit for what appears to be a permanent cure of cancer—a cancer that is 95 percent fatal in most similar cases.

To give credit where credit is due, the Schmidts arranged a public Mass of Thanksgiving for the healing of Roell Ann on August 23 [1976] at St. Roch Church. . . . Some 80 persons attended, most of them persons who had been praying fervently for Roell's recovery for nearly a year. . . .

David Schmidt, 34, a history teacher by training, and his wife, Barbara, 38, an English professor at Southern Illinois University, Edwardsville, have been parishioners at St. Roch for all 10 years of their marriage. They have a son, Karl, now 9, but it was a urinary infection in their second child, Roell, that first caused concern back in June, 1975. It was the second such infection in 10 months, and the Schmidts were advised to get a special X-ray examination.

On July 28, 1975, just after Roell's third birthday, X-rays taken at St. Louis Children's Hospital disclosed that Roell's internal organs seemed normal, but that a three-centimeter calcified mass was located near her adrenal gland, on her right side. There was 99 percent likelihood the mass was a benign tumor, the doctors said, but [they] recommended surgery as soon as possible to make certain, and to remove it.

The news started Mrs. Schmidt to worrying—and the fear and doubt that followed led her to prayer, "mainly because I just couldn't stand it anymore." Within weeks she began attending the Wednesday evening meetings of the St. Roch Parish Prayer Group.

After several delays caused by infections, exploratory surgery was finally performed on Sept. 9, 1975, by the team of surgical specialists at St. Louis Children's Hospital.

The results were devastating. What was thought to be a benign tumor was, in fact, 100 percent malignant cancer; moreover, cancerous cells were spread throughout the adrenal and lymph glands so extensively as to be inoperable. It was, said Dr. Vita Land, a stage III neuroblastoma. In infants under age one, such tumors sometimes dissolved on their own. But in someone of Roell's age, the doctor reported grimly, it was 95 percent fatal. There was only a 50-50 chance of prolonging

Roell's life for any time at all, the doctor added, provided they began radiation and drug therapies.

Intense radiation therapies began almost immediately. So did the Schmidts' intense prayer. "Why? Because I'm a fighter," Mrs. Schmidt said firmly, "and David is, too. We began asking anyone—everyone—to pray." They solicited the prayer of David's mother's south side prayer group, nuns in Sioux City, Jesuits at St. Louis U., the Benedictine Nuns on Morgantown Rd., even Grace Methodist Church, just down the street from St. Roch Church.

Following 20 days of intense radiation, Roell began a projected 18- to 24-month series of drug therapy. The Schmidts were referred in October to another prayer resource, as well—Merton House, the residence of Father Francis MacNutt, O.P.*

"Father MacNutt said he had no hesitation about praying for the healing of a child," Mrs. Schmidt related. "In fact, he said the chances for success were pretty good."

Thus, every Thursday afternoon, the Schmidts brought Roell to Merton House. Sometimes with Father MacNutt, sometimes just with his associate, Sister Mary Margaret McKenzie, V.H.M., or with others who were on hand, they would pray that God would heal Roell of cancer.

The sessions would last about 30 minutes, Mrs. Schmidt related. They would begin by Father MacNutt placing his hands on Roell's right side approximately where the tumor was located. There was often a brief anointing with blessed oil, on the youngster's forehead and also at the site of the tumor. Then would come a period of prayer aloud. "Sometimes he would appeal for God to heal the tumor; sometimes for a change in symptoms; or for the relief from the side effects of the drug therapy. . . ." Others present who were inclined would also pray for the little girl. Then all would recite the Our Father in unison. The session would conclude with Roell leading the singing of "Everybody All Love Jesus," a nursery hymn she had learned.

---

*Since this article was written, Francis MacNutt has left the priesthood and is now the director of Christian Healing Ministries, P.O. Box 9520, Jacksonville, FL 32208.

At first, the Schmidts were just silent participants. "It took me three months before I was confident enough to join aloud in the prayers," Mrs. Schmidt said. . . .

Shortly after the Merton House sessions began, Father MacNutt administered to Roell the Sacrament of the Anointing of the Sick. Earlier that fall it had been given by an associate pastor of their parish. (By the time it was all over, Roell would have received some two dozen blessings with oil, although not all were the complete rite of the sacrament.)

From the beginning, the Schmidts were touched by the Merton House sessions. "Right away, the experience seemed to uplift us," David Schmidt said, and Barbara elaborated. "We felt like we had come on a pilgrimage. . . . The quality of the prayer seemed so intense and so deep. It really seemed to cut through to the heart of the matter."

In November, a small event occurred which struck the Schmidts deeply.

"One morning when I was doing the ironing," Mrs. Schmidt related; "Roell came out of her bedroom and said: 'Mommy, God says you're gonna get well.'

"'Oh,' I replied, 'I didn't know I was sick.'

"'No,' she told me, sort of irritated, 'God meant that I'm gonna get well.'"

Mrs. Schmidt related the exchange that evening to her husband, who was struck by the child's use of the pronoun "you" as if the girl was repeating exactly what she had heard.

"Neither of us dared to believe it," Mrs. Schmidt continued, "but we did take some comfort from it. And it buoyed us over a very bad time."

The times were bad, indeed. The radiation caused Roell to lose most of her hair—a common consequence—and the drug therapies were having their own severe side effect on the three-year-old: she would lose her appetite, blood counts would drop, she became feverish and caught a number of viral infections. The drugs were suspended to relieve the side effects, then the treatment cycle would be resumed.

As 1976 began, there were plans for a second exploratory surgery, to see how much good the treatments were doing, but the plans were dropped. Roell seemed to be "holding her own," the doctors related, and they recommended that the therapies be continued.

The Schmidts continued praying: Wednesday nights with the parish prayer group; Thursday afternoons at Morton House, accompanied by Roell.

In late May, the team at Children's Hospital decided that if the drug therapies were allowed to continue, there would be permanent damage to Roell's heart, and that the time had come for surgery to both assess the effect of the treatments and to remove as much of the cancerous tumor as possible.

On June 22, the surgery was performed by Dr. Lawrence O'Neal at Children's Hospital, in which he removed the still-existing calcified mass, one-third of the adrenal gland and four lymph glands. The Schmidts—and, by then, their hundreds of allies—were praying intensely.

Three days later, June 25, the doctors gave the laboratory report to the Schmidts as follows:

- the tumor was found to have zero cancer cells;

- the other glands were not only free of malignancy, but were found to possess a number of ganglion, i.e., healthy growing nerve tissue cells;

- that while the therapies may have halted the cancer cells, the medical team could not claim any credit for the appearance or growth of these healthy cells;

- such a turnaround, in patients of similar age and condition, was so very uncommon as to be remarkable.

"We were so numb from weariness and anxiety that it took a week for the news to really sink in," Mrs. Schmidt said. They promptly told Father MacNutt.

"He was thrilled, and does feel that he and the others have been God's instrument," she said.

David Schmidt, after long reflection and thought about it, attributes Roell's apparent cure this way:

"There is no doubt that prayer—especially the prayer at Merton House with Father MacNutt and Sister Mary Margaret and those with the St. Roch prayer group—have brought this about. But neither am I ready to say that the radiation and the drug therapies were unnecessary.

"We don't have medical evidence that a miracle occurred," he continued. "But neither do we have evidence that the therapies effected the cell differentiation, the cure. Who knows? Maybe someday they'll discover how this differentiation occurs.

"All I know for sure is that God cured our daughter. Whether it was through the efforts of the team at Children's Hospital or whether the malignant cells just disappeared, is a moot question."

Dr. Land calls it "the $64,000 question," but has the same assessment. "We're not sure what caused the change; all I know is that in 95 percent of the cases, the child is dead in two years."

Mrs. Schmidt adds a second blessing. "The quality of their prayer at Morton House buoyed us from week to week. Without it, our family would never have survived," she said. This is not a minor victory, she noted, inasmuch as cancer in children has an almost malevolent effect on the parents. Children's Hospital has a social worker to treat family stress among cases of children's cancer, they related.

Since June, the Schmidts have continued their weekly prayer sessions. For one thing, Roell is almost 100 percent certain to have been sterilized by the intense radiation treatments. "We pray that God, having cured her, does not allow her to perish as a result of the side effects," David Schmidt noted.

Moreover, Roell can give very encouraging witness to other cancer patients, and the Schmidts themselves feel a desire to pray for others, especially for cancer victims.

They scheduled the Aug. 23 Mass at St. Roch in order to give public thanks to God for Roell's cure, they noted, and plan to continue their prayer—now a prayer of thanks.

"I've prayed for healing," David Schmidt observed, "and I've prayed for thanks—and, believe me, it's much nicer to give thanks."

Postscript: Roell graduated from college and is still free of cancer.

Landy's Story

Anne Ponder, who wrote this account for us, is a mother of two grown children and lives in Griffin, Georgia. We learned of her son, Landy, through Francis MacNutt.

My son Landy had always been an extremely healthy, athletic young man. He played Junior Varsity basketball in the ninth and tenth grades and then made the varsity team in his junior year. But soon afterward he began to lose his strength and realized that he could not stay on the team. He also started losing facial hair, which greatly embarrassed him. At the beginning of Landy's senior year, I noticed that he was extremely thirsty all the time. Though he and a friend won all their matches of doubles tennis until they reached the regional finals, Landy was still not up to par. We had him tested for diabetes by two different doctors, but neither doctor could find anything wrong.

After his freshman year at Auburn, Landy came home to work at a summer job. He was still very thirsty and often tired after work. When he went back to start his sophomore year, his abnormal thirst continued. Now he began to lose weight. When his grades started to fall, Landy left school and came home to get a job in Hampton. While he was home I was able to watch him more closely. I insisted he go to Emory Clinic in Atlanta to see an endocrinologist recommended by our family doctor.

In July 1986, Landy was examined by Dr. Richard V. Clark at Emory. A week later Dr. Clark called: "Mrs. Ponder, I have reason to believe your son has a brain tumor."

The only words I heard were BRAIN TUMOR. It is impossible to describe the shock. All I could feel was panic. I had worried for years that Landy might have a car wreck, but never had I imagined anything like this. The entire summer was spent having MRIs [pictures taken by a radiologist; these are described in chapter 3] and other tests, seeing various doctors and adjusting hormone dosages. The next month (August 1986), Landy was put into the hospital to determine the correct dosage for a drug to regulate his fluid balance. By fall, the supplemental hormones had added over forty pounds to his frame. All I can remember is buying many different sizes of clothes during those months.

Because my husband and I believe that God still heals today, we asked for a healing service at our church. Landy was open to this. With many of our friends in attendance, our minister anointed Landy with oil and the group prayed for him. Landy said that while his eyes were closed in prayer he could see a cross with light all around it.

In September 1986, Landy returned to Auburn with the knowledge that he would have to be checked regularly to see if the tumor had started to grow. He hoped it would not grow because he knew that the treatment for a growing tumor would be dreadful. On December 23, Dr. Clark gave us the bad news: the tumor seemed to be growing, so Landy might have to have a brain biopsy.

Landy was right to be worried. The brain biopsy, performed in the spring of 1987, was absolute torture. The surgery required that Landy remain awake while the surgeon opened his skull and put a needle into the center of his brain to take a biopsy of the tumor. Screws were placed into his scalp and tightened so that Landy could not move. His head felt like it would burst. Landy called the doctor every name he knew to call him.

We waited for eight hours during the surgery; finally, the doctor came. He told us that he thought it was a mixed germ-cell tumor on the hypothalmus, but that it might be something else. Even after the brain tumor board met to discuss the case, there still seemed to be some uncertainty about the diagnosis.

Then we learned that Dr. Abdel Ragab, head of pediatric hematology, wanted to begin chemotherapy right away. In the first week of May, he met with us to present his plan. We told him that the Lord is the healer, so Dr. Ragab would have more help than usual with this young man. Dr. Ragab replied, "We don't care who gets the credit."

About a year before this time, I had listened to some tapes from a seminar for health professionals at which Francis and Judith MacNutt* had spoken. After listening to the tapes again, I was convinced that we needed to take Landy to Francis to be prayed for.

After several frantic phone calls, I reached the MacNutts in their home in Jacksonville, Florida. Judith MacNutt advised us to ask for prayer from as many people as possible from as large a geographic area as possible. So we called our friends who were believers from Texas to Florida, and from Washington to Maryland. (We later discovered that people we didn't even know were praying for Landy.)

After doing all that we knew to do, we felt we also needed to come to someone who we felt had a gift of healing. So we made arrangements to fly to Jacksonville on the following Monday to see the MacNutts and to get prayer for Landy on Tuesday.

But we were also supposed to start chemotherapy with Dr. Ragab on the same Tuesday, so I called to change the appointment. I felt sure that Dr. Ragab would object; he had been concerned about starting the treatments as soon as possible. To my surprise, Dr. Ragab's secretary told me that he had been suddenly called out of the country to see his mother, who was sick in Egypt. God's timing was amazing!

On Monday we flew to Jacksonville, where Landy was prayed for by Francis MacNutt and a group of precious people on his staff. Then, as soon as we returned home, we got back on the plane to see Dr. Roger Packer in Philadelphia. (Dr. Packer was one of the two doctors in the country at the time who were doing research on germ-cell tumors.) All of this activity in a week's time—we had to ship Landy's X-rays and records by overnight express to Philadelphia—made our heads swim, but we sensed God was doing something. A day after he was prayed for, Landy's double vision (which he had had for four months) went away.

I felt sure, after this sign, that Landy was healed. Dr. Packer confirmed Landy's original diagnosis (mixed germ-cell tumor) but recommended that more tests be done before treatment began. I was excited— sure that these tests would show that Landy was healed!

They didn't. The long ordeal of chemotherapy was about to begin. Dr. Packer told us to have Dr. Ragab wait for the new protocol [prescription of chemotherapy drugs] for germ-cell tumor treatment. He said it was tougher at the beginning, but probably more effective—the old procedure was successful for only 10 percent of patients.

---

*By this time, Francis MacNutt had left the priesthood and had married.

At that point I could see God's direction in all that was happening. If Dr. Ragab had not been unexpectedly called to Egypt, Landy might not have gotten the prayer, and Dr. Ragab might have used the old, less successful protocol. I sensed that God was leading us to proceed with the medical procedures and continue to trust in him.

The protocol was tough—five days of intravenous chemotherapy, three weeks off for the blood to restore itself, then five more days, and so on for a period of four months. At the end of the second treatment, we were to have a CAT scan [see chapter 3 for an explanation of this test] done to see if the tumor had grown. If it had, Landy would have to go straight to radiation therapy.

Much to Dr. Ragab's surprise, on 19 July 1987, the CAT-scan report showed—no tumor! When he called, he said, "Mrs. Ponder, you will not believe this."

"Oh, yes I will," I replied. "Try me."

"It is gone. The tumor is completely gone."

"It's the Lord," I said. "We told you we were going to have some extra help, Dr. Ragab."

"Yes, I know, and I believe, but I have never seen anything like this. The tumor is completely gone. I had to go to the radiologist's and see for myself. That is why I am so late calling."

Dr. Ragab said that he wanted to continue with the protocol for fear that the tumor might return. I felt sorry for Landy. Believing that God had healed him made a continuation of the chemotherapy that much harder on him. He, his dad, and I cried together one afternoon on the hospital patio before the third round of treatments began, but we made it through the third and fourth rounds of chemotherapy. Then came radiation.

The next six weeks were grueling. We drove up to Emory every day, and Landy was sick all the way back. I spent my time trying to build his blood back up by feeding him calf liver and fresh carrots cooked crisply with fresh parsley and lemon juice. Landy spent many hours on the den sofa. He lost his hair again for the third time.

We finally finished radiation on 27 November 1987. He returned to Auburn University and graduated in December 1991. It's been five years since he completed radiation, and the tumor is still gone. (He has had checkups and CAT scans regularly to confirm this.) In fact, after a checkup in July 1992, Dr. Ragab proclaimed, "I don't think the tumor will come back if it hasn't already. I consider you cured!" We've been elated ever since.

Landy feels well; he enjoys hunting, fishing, tennis, and golf when he is not teaching fourth grade in his hometown. He needs to take thyroid and cortisone replacements and may have to take hormones the rest of his life. (I'm praying that God will heal what was damaged so he can stop taking those things.) But Landy is alive and well, and we're grateful!

Postscript: In 1997, Landy was married, teaching third grade, working on his master's degree, and enjoying hunting whatever is in season.

Joan's Story

Joan McDermott,* a mother of seven grown children, lives in the Chicago area with her husband. The following is her own account of her experience with cancer.

I first discovered that I had a serious problem in May of 1977. It was a week before my second son's wedding; we were at Cape Cod on vacation. One night I noticed that I had a lump in my abdomen. I thought it was a hernia.

As soon as I got back from vacation I went to see my doctor. She knew immediately that the lump was a tumor, and she arranged an appointment with a surgeon for the following day. The surgeon confirmed my doctor's suspicion and arranged for surgery the following week. When I woke up after surgery, I was told that I had ovarian cancer. The doctors had taken a cancerous tumor the size of a grapefruit out of my abdomen. They had also found malignant nodules on the underside

---

*Gerry's mother.

of my liver but had left them alone. They told my husband that at the end of one year, seven out of ten women in my condition would be dead, and at the end of two years, at least one more would have died.

I was shocked—and scared. But I shouldn't have been shocked. Two of my sisters had already died from bone cancer, and another had recovered from cancer. And in 1974, three years before my cancer was discovered, I had had another scare. Margaret, my fourth sister, had been taken into surgery for uterine cancer. In desperation I told my church friends, who gathered to pray with me for her. One person in the group felt led to pray against a curse of cancer on my family. I was deeply moved by that prayer and sensed that something really had happened in the spiritual realm. As it turned out, Margaret fully recovered and has had no recurrence of cancer in the twenty-three years since.

When I learned that I had cancer, I remembered Margaret's recovery and that stirring prayer, and I felt that perhaps now my faith in God was being tested and tried. At the same time, I had all the normal reactions to the news of cancer—fear of the future, fear of dying, anxiety over what would happen to my husband, my three teenagers still at home, and my four grown children.

The most comforting and encouraging words came from my pastor, who visited me in the hospital. He came to see me the day after I got the news of cancer and gave me many wonderful Bible passages—each one written out on an index card for me to meditate on:

> My times are in your hands.
> When I am afraid, I will trust in you.
> In God, whose word I praise, in God I trust;
> I will not be afraid.
> Praise the LORD . . .
> who forgives all your sins and heals all your diseases.
> He sent forth his word and healed them.
> He was pierced for our transgressions,
> he was crushed for our iniquities;
> the punishment that brought us peace was upon him,
> and by his wounds we are healed.[23]

These passages spoke straight to my heart. Meditating on them began to produce in me faith and hope that God could heal me. I began to have faith that my life was in God's loving hands and that he would take care of me, regardless of the outcome. Yet for a while it was hard to hang on to this hope because everyone around me thought I was going to die. My doctors were convinced that it was just a question of how many months I had left. And my husband and most of my children were so devastated by the doctors' reports that they seemed resigned to losing me.

But then my second son, Sean, came to see me from Wyoming. He came into my room on a bright sunny day, kissed me and held me, and then announced with tears in his eyes, "Mom, I believe God is going to heal you."

With these words, a dam in my heart broke, and all of the pent-up emotion burst forth in a flood of tears. I cried, but with tears of relief.

"Oh, Sean, you're the first one who has any hope! Everyone else has given me up for dead!" I sobbed.

Sean and I prayed together. He prayed, with confidence and deep emotion, that God would dry up the cancer in my abdomen. From that day forward, my faith grew.

Sean talked to his father and sisters, persuading them to pray and believe that I would be healed. He also talked to my church. Pretty soon my other son, Richard, who was newly married, came over with his wife every Monday night to pray for me. Friends from church committed themselves to coming to our home to pray for me every week for two years. I was "soaked" with prayer for healing.

After reading some books on healing, we all became convinced that sick people need more prayer than the usual one time of laying on of hands. They need the continual loving prayers of a committed group of people. It was these repeated doses of prayer—twice every week as family and friends laid their hands on me to pray—that helped my faith and trust in God to deepen. I believe it was this soaking prayer that also healed me.

I took chemotherapy pills for five months but decided on my own [with input from her doctor] to stop taking them. When I saw that my white blood cell count was too high and my red blood cell count too low, I decided to end the treatments.

I can truly say that I never experienced pain after my surgery, and after a year I had regained my former strength. Two years after the operation I had another liver scan to see what had happened to those cancerous nodules on my liver. To my joy, they had done nothing! I followed through with six-month checkups for two years and then annual checkups at five years, six years, and so on. No sign of cancer has ever again appeared! In February of 1997 it was twenty years since I was diagnosed with ovarian cancer.

The nurse in my doctor's office one time confided in me that the staff was intrigued by my case. Although my doctor at my ten-year checkup would not agree with me that God had intervened, she seemed pleased and awed that I was alive and well.

How Do I Pray for Healing?

Perhaps you have cancer or have a loved one with cancer and want to pray for healing. Where do you start? How do you do it? In this last part of this chapter we will share some guidelines that may prove helpful.

There Is No One Method

The first thing to know is that there is no one sure-fire method of healing prayer that should always be followed. Jesus rarely prayed in the same way twice. Many times he healed simply by speaking a word to a person, yet the words were often different. To a paralyzed man, for example, he said, "Get up, take your mat and go home." (At that, Matthew records, the man simply "got up and went home.") To a leper he simply said, "Be clean!"[24]

On many other occasions, Jesus used physical touch to impart his healing power. He touched the hand of Peter's mother-in-law who had a fever, the eyes of two blind men to restore their sight, and the ear of the high priest's servant after it had been sliced off. He "took hold" of a man with dropsy, "put his hands on" a crippled woman, and took the hand of Jairus' daughter to raise her from the dead. One time his merely touching the coffin of a widow's son was enough to bring the boy back to life.[25]

But Jesus was not restricted to words or a simple touch. To heal the man born blind, Jesus spit on the ground, made mud with the saliva, and daubed some of the mud on the man's eyes. For another blind man he used saliva alone, spitting on the man's eyes and putting his hands on him. On several other occasions, people got well merely by putting their hands on him.[26]

The lesson to be learned from this brief examination of Jesus' healing methods in the Gospels is that you shouldn't be too concerned with the way you pray as long as you pray!

Physical touch conveys the warmth of love, which cancer patients need to receive as much as anyone. It was a practice Jesus often used to impart his healing power—but it was not the only practice. We suggest that you pray in a manner that is most comfortable to you and the person receiving prayer. Many Christians, following the biblical admonition in James 5, anoint the sick person with oil when they pray.

Deal with Attitudes That Block Healing

Far more important than the physical mode of prayer is the attitude of heart. One attitude that prevents some cancer victims from receiving prayer is a sense of unworthiness. "Healing is for saints," they say, "and I'm no saint."

Besides missing the biblical assumption that all believers are saints,[27] this statement also implies that God gives his gifts (such as healing) only to those who deserve it. But this flies in the face of the overriding message of the Bible—that God loves the unlovable and pours out his gifts on those who don't deserve them.

In fact, the Bible teaches that every one of us is unworthy of God's gifts. This means that those who think they are worthy are truly unworthy. They are self-righteous, unaware of the corruption that actually lives in their hearts. As such, they are outside of the kingdom of God, whose residents, according to Jesus, are "poor in spirit"—that is, they recognize their spiritual poverty. So the feeling of being unworthy makes one, in a sense, worthy of the gift of healing![28]

Those who have been engaged in ministries of healing also report that unforgiveness is a common block in preventing healing. In his superb study of the healing ministry, Francis MacNutt wrote:

> The key form of repentance we need is to forgive our enemies. I have found that many sins do not block God's healing power to the same extent as does a lack of forgiveness. I understand better than I used to why Jesus laid such a heavy stress on forgiving enemies when he talked about prayer. He doesn't talk nearly as much about drunkenness and lust as he does about being unforgiving. Furthermore, he often seems to connect forgiving enemies with the Father's answering our prayers:
>
> > I tell you therefore: everything you ask and pray for, believe that you have it already, and it will be yours. And when you stand in prayer, forgive whatever you have against anybody, so that your Father in heaven may forgive your failings too. (Mark 11:24–25)
>
> I used to consider such passages as a kind of jumping from one subject to another: in one sentence Jesus enjoins faith in prayer; in the next he enjoins us to forgive. But now I see that the two ideas are intimately connected. It's as if God's saving, healing, forgiving love cannot flow into us unless we are ready to let it flow to others. If we deny forgiveness and healing to others, God's love cannot flow into us. It's all part of the great commandment in which loving our neighbor is part of the same commandment as loving God. "I love God only as much as I love my worst enemy." There is a direct relationship between our willingness to love others and the healing ministry.[29]

After Jesus' death, the early church continued to connect confession of sins such as unforgiveness with healing. James wrote, for instance, "Confess your sins to each other and pray for each other so that you may be healed."[30]

The implications of this for the cancer patient are clear. If you seek healing power from God, you should search your heart for unforgiveness or bitterness, confess these attitudes as sin, and ask for divine help to forgive.

Pray with Faith

Although Jesus sometimes healed people who had little or no involvement in the transformation, most healings in his ministry and the early church came as the result of someone's faith in God. Jesus frequently said after healing someone, "Your faith has healed you." When Paul saw a crippled man in Lystra, he "looked directly at him, *saw that he had faith to be healed* and called out, 'Stand up on your feet!'" After healing a crippled beggar in Jerusalem, Peter told the onlookers, "By faith in the name of Jesus, this man whom you see and know was made strong. It is Jesus' name *and the faith that comes through him* that has given this complete healing to him, as you can all see."[31]

Faith, then, was an important element in most of the healings recorded in the New Testament. But *faith* is a slippery word; it means different things to different people. What was the sort of faith that the early Christians had that enabled them to be healed? What is the faith that Roell's parents had—and Landy's mother, and Joan McDermott?

It is difficult to state clearly what healing faith is; it is easier to say what it is *not*. For instance, it is clear from the healing testimonies of people both two thousand years ago and today that the faith that heals is not faith in faith. In other words, these people did not place their confidence in the power of their belief to somehow destroy their diseases. They were not counting on their own positive thinking or their own supposedly divine potential to cure themselves. Instead, they placed their confidence in the living God.

Healing faith is also not the same as the certainty that healing will occur. People who have healing faith are often very aware they do not know all of the factors involved in a given situation. God may want to heal. On the other hand, God alone may know some factor that may make it better for the person *not* to be healed. God answers our prayers for healing, but sometimes his answer may be no.

Healing faith recognizes that healing is ultimately a mystery hidden from mortal minds. As Francis MacNutt wrote:

> Healing is mysterious. The best that man can do is to bow down before the mystery that is God. When God chooses to reveal his mind, we can act with assurance. At other times, when we are in doubt about a particular case, the most honest thing to do is to admit the doubt and bow down before the mystery.[32]

Healing faith, then, is not faith in faith, and it is not certainty of healing. But then what is it? We can say on the basis of the biblical record, the teachings of the Judeo-Christian tradition, and the experience of those who have experienced healing, *that healing faith is trust in God's love, leaving the results up to him.* Healing faith involves praying for God to heal while trusting that he will do what is best, whether it be healing or something else. As Joan wrote, "I began to have faith that my life was in God's loving hands and that he would take care of me, *regardless of the outcome.*"[33]

Leaving the results to God does not mean that we don't know whether God will answer our prayer. Sometimes people pray for healing and add, "If it be your will," as if doubting that God will answer the prayer.

The faith we are describing prays instead, "Let this be done according to your will," with the full assurance that God will answer the prayer in his own wise manner.

Improper understandings of faith have led to much heartache and bitterness. Mike, a man in his late fifties, believed that God would heal him. When in his last months it became apparent that he was dying, he stubbornly refused to consider the possibility that it was not God's will for him to be healed. The result was that both he and his family were shocked and unprepared when he died. Some of the family, we fear, may still be bitter toward God because Mike was not physically healed.

Mike's mistake was his refusal to consider the possibility that cancer might be God's way of taking him home to himself. So he denied that he was dying, even while his body filled with fluids and needed extraordinary medical means to keep breathing. As a result, he may have caused lasting spiritual problems for his family.

David Watson almost made that same mistake. John Wimber and his ministry teams flew to London to pray repeatedly for David's healing for hours at a time. But eventually it became clear that his condition was steadily worsening. In John's words:

> Fluids continued to collect in his body; I knew he was dying. I could hardly look at him, I loved him so much.
>
> One day toward the end of his visit I had a long, frank conversation with him. Up to that time he had still been making plans for the coming year as though he were not ill. "David," I said, "you're a dying man, and you're denying it."
>
> "I know," he said.
>
> "Unless God sovereignly intervenes, you will die," I said. "Go home and get your affairs in good order. Your faith in Christ has been a constant source of encouragement to me. But you have to acknowledge that you are dying."
>
> David said that, whether his health improved or not, his trust in God would not be shaken.[34]

David Watson died in peace and in faith. Just as the biblical heroes of faith "were all commended for their faith, yet none of them received what had been promised,"[35] so Watson maintained his faith even though he was not physically healed. He recognized God's sovereignty—God's freedom to heal some and not heal others, while answering all prayers for healing with what is best, in love.

Use "Soaking Prayer"

A final guideline to consider when seeking healing is the notion of "soaking prayer." This is the practice that Francis MacNutt described at length in *The Power to Heal* and that was used in both Roell's and Joan's healings. The basic idea is that just as the ground is better watered by repeated soakings of rain than by one sudden downpour, healing seems to come more often and effectively after or through repeated applications of gentle, loving prayer.

Many believers have been taught that we are to pray only once for healing—that repeated prayer only betrays lack of faith in God's power or beneficence. Does God need to be asked more than once, it is sometimes asked, to do what is good? Don't we believe that God can hear us the first time? Yet we also know that God can heal without any prayer at all. So healing after only one prayer is itself an example of God's accommodation to our finite capacities.

Theologians have often said that God chooses to do certain things (such as heal) in response to prayer in order to teach human beings their dependence on him. While he could just as easily act without hearing human prayer, he has chosen to act in response to prayer in order to draw his people closer to himself. In this sense, answers to prayer are instances of God's stooping to accommodate himself to our finite capacities. If answered prayer itself is an example of God's accommodation to our finite capacities, then God's waiting to heal until repeated prayers are made or his gradual healing through repeated prayer, can be seen simply as an extension of this principle.

We see examples of soaking prayer in the Bible. In the Garden of Gethsemane, Jesus had to pray not once, but three times on the same subject before he could come to clarity of mind and heart. Paul had to pray not once but three times about his thorn in the flesh before God answered his prayer. After Jesus prayed for a blind man to be healed, the man still had blurry vision. Only after Jesus prayed a second time was the man's sight fully restored.[36] MacNutt and others argue that if Jesus and Paul had to pray more than once for some of their prayers to be answered, why should we have to limit ourselves to once?

We believe that soaking prayer has another benefit for cancer patients; it helps them feel the ongoing love and support of other people. Roell, Landy, Joan, and others were reassured of their friends' love for them by their repeated prayers, and this reaffirmation of love—expressed through prayer—buoyed their faith.

Healing Is Possible

In conclusion, we believe that healing is possible today. God does not always choose to heal—or he chooses to heal in ways other than physical. But sometimes, for his own mysterious reasons, God does show his love and compassion by physically healing some of cancer. Prayer for healing is a way for us to exercise faith and show love for those who are fighting cancer.

If you have difficulty knowing what to pray, you may want to use part or all of the following prayer:

> Father God, I choose to believe that you are the same yesterday, today, and forever. I believe that you healed people in the Bible, that you have healed people in history since then, and that you are still healing people today. You are all-powerful. For you, cancer is very easy to heal, if you so choose. And your love and compassion for your people is very great.
>
> God, I confess to you that I have fallen far short of your demands for my life. I have sinned in thought, word, and deed. I have not given you the thanks and praise that you deserve, nor have I treated my family and neighbors with the love they deserve. Show me, God, if I have an unforgiving heart. Give me the grace to forgive those who have wounded me. Show me if there is any other bad attitude or habit in me that you want me to deal with.
>
> Thank you, Lord, that you are a God of forgiveness and compassion. Thank you, too, for being a God who loves to bless the unworthy. I ask you to send your supernatural power to destroy my cancer. I believe that you work through doctors and medicine, and I pray that you will fill the doctors and nurses and technicians who work on my case with wisdom and love. But I also ask you to do what doctors and medicine cannot do. In your mercy, immobilize and paralyze the cancerous cells in my body that medicine cannot reach. Dry up whatever is feeding those cells with life. Put a stop to the spread of cancer in my body.
>
> God, I trust that you will do whatever is best for me. If it is your will, you will heal me. Give me the strength and ability to keep trusting in

that truth. And if I am not healed, please give me the power to trust you then too. But most important of all, bring me closer to you. Open my eyes and my heart so that I may come to a deeper experience of your love for me. Help me to do whatever is necessary to draw closer to you and to know you as my heavenly Father. AMEN.

14

Why Not Suicide?

Another Look at the Kevorkian Approach

Not long ago Bill treated a man who had come to the emergency room because of constipation. The constipation was an indirect result of cancer; his pain pills and poor diet had led to dehydration, which in turn produced constipation. After a nurse had disimpacted the man and Bill had told him what he should do to ensure it didn't happen again, the patient headed for the door. But just before exiting the room, he turned to Bill and smiled. "Nice knowing you, doc." Bill sensed that this man was eager for conversation.

"What do you have planned for today?" Bill asked, trying to get something started. The man replied that he was going to get his affairs in order. Before too long he confessed to Bill that he planned to kill himself. The gun was loaded in the garage, and a noose had already been secured to the rafters. So if the gun didn't do the job, the noose would.

The real problem, then, was not constipation but an impatience to die. Bill asked the man if anyone was helping him at home, what medicines he had for his discomfort, and when the home health care nurse had visited him last. His invalid wife, none, and never were his answers.

So Bill told him about hospice: the volunteer who will do almost anything, the medicines that are provided for many uncomfortable symptoms of cancer, and the nurse who visits regularly.

"Well, I guess that changes my plans," the man replied. He then agreed to talk to a hospice worker. Eventually he entered hospice and died, but not at his own hand and only after several more rewarding months with his loved ones.

The hospice option is a side of the debate over physician-assisted suicide that often goes unheard (see the next chapter). It is drowned out by the publicity surrounding Dr. Jack Kevorkian, who gives the impression that his way is the only way to die with dignity.

Modern medicine's phenomenal ability to prolong life has made Kevorkian seem credible. Technology is now available to extend the dying process to often unbearable extents. Our doctors have been trained to save lives at any cost. As a result, we are living longer and longer.

Families are changing too. Both spouses often work (which leaves no one at home to care for the dying), the extended family rarely lives in the same household, and most of us in the last two generations have neither seen someone die nor cared for a dying loved one in our homes. So we're caught between a rock and a hard place. Dying at home seems logistically impossible, and dying in a hospital seems both humiliating and excruciating. We're afraid of being subjected to some maniac doctor who never gives up, never gives in, and never gives morphine. And the thought of being a burden on our families, either financially or emotionally, makes the prospect of dying even more frightening. It's no wonder that Kevorkian's approach is appealing to many.

A Disturbing Trend

Situations like these have persuaded an increasing number of Americans to consider as a viable option physician-assisted suicide—a procedure that until very recently was illegal in all fifty states. More and more Americans seem to believe that it should be legal. In November 1994, for example, Oregon voters narrowly approved Measure 16, which gives doctors freedom to prescribe lethal drugs to patients who appear to have less than six months to live. In the spring of 1996, the Ninth Circuit Court of Appeals (with jurisdiction over California, Alaska, Arizona, Hawaii, Idaho, Montana, Nevada, Oregon, and Washington)[1] and the Second Circuit Court of Appeals (with jurisdiction over New York, Connecticut, and Vermont)[2] both struck down state laws forbidding physician-assisted suicide.

Some Americans favor even involuntary euthanasia. That is, they support the administration of a lethal drug by a doctor to terminally or chronically ill patients without their consent. In a disturbing recent poll, 90 percent of one group of economics students supported involuntary euthanasia for unspecified groups of people to "streamline the economy."[3]

Why are more Americans coming to support a practice that until not so long ago was condemned by nearly all? In this chapter we will look at four arguments that are commonly given by those who support physician-assisted suicide. Not all of them are directly related to cancer, but all bear some relation to the underlying attitudes that cancer patients and their families share when they consider suicide.

I Don't Want Heroic Measures to Prolong My Dying

I remember my friend Harold, a godly and mature Christian who died of cancer ten years ago. As he lay dying, he told me, "I don't fear death, but I do fear dying." Like many of us, he was afraid of endless medical procedures that would be both expensive and painful. He just wanted to go home to be with his Lord, and he didn't want his dying prolonged artificially by heroic and extraordinary measures.

It was not always like this. Before the rise of modern medicine, people most often died at home. By 1950, 50 percent of all Americans died in hospitals. Now 80 percent die there—often separated from the loved ones they most need in their last hours. Why are so many subjected to what seems to be "cruel and unusual punishment" at the time when they need not technology but our love? There are many reasons:

1. Some families believe that earthly life is all there is, so even another day is worth further procedures.

2. Some Christians stubbornly cling to the hope of healing, even when death is on the doorstep, and believe that they would fail in faith if they didn't ask doctors to do everything possible.

3. Distant relatives feel guilty about not having been more available when the patient was well and don't see the suffering that heroic measures often involve, so they demand that the doctor "do everything."

4. Others fear they could not afford the expenses of bringing their dying loved one home.

5. Some patients and their families don't realize they can refuse more treatment.

6. Some doctors fear that failing to cure their patients also means they have failed as doctors.

7. Other doctors are afraid of being sued if they don't do everything possible to keep a patient breathing. As a result, the art of caring for the dying has given way to an art of maintaining the heartbeat at all cost.[4]

But Christians need to be encouraged that there is nothing wrong with permitting their loved one to die when it is clear that the dying process has begun. Extraordinary and heroic measures to keep the patient breathing just a bit longer are not always best for the patient and may only prolong artificially the process that has begun to bring God's child home. "There is a time to die," Scripture tells us.[5] When the patient's condition and a trusted physician tell us that this time has come, we need not feel guilty about refusing or withdrawing treatment beyond helping the patient feel comfortable.

Even intravenous food and water at times can be unpleasant and burdensome to the patient, and only prolong the dying process. Sustenance should be offered to all dying patients, but if patients refuse, their wishes should be honored. Bill has had many conversations about this with well-intentioned loved ones who have a very difficult time understanding this. He asks them to try to recall the last time they overate. Perhaps it was a third helping of lasagna, he jokes. Or perhaps they remember the wave of nausea that came over them when their host urged them to have another piece of cheesecake.

Bill explains that many cancer patients feel that discomfort or nausea much of the day. While the need for food seems obvious to us, the act of eating seems impossible to some patients, and sometimes it is. Distaste for food and eating is part of the dying process; a patient's refusal to eat should be honored.

This is very different from physician-assisted suicide or euthanasia. In the process I have just described, there is an underlying fatal pathology that is inexorably leading to death. But physician-assisted suicide and euthanasia provide their own pathologies. This is the difference (a critical and oft-neglected difference in today's debate over physician-assisted suicide) between allowing to die, on the one hand, and killing, on the other. We are permitted by God to allow ourselves or our loved ones to die without extraordinary measures, but we are not permitted to kill.

Perhaps we can illustrate this difference by comparing human life to the flight of a plane. Imagine an old airplane that is having engine trouble and is flying through a bad storm. Its engine may have flown too many miles and reached the point where no amount of repair work will ever get it flying again. Now, during this flight, something has popped in the engine. It continues to function, and with patience and care it can be landed gently. But it will never be able to take off again.

When the body is dying of cancer, it is like that airplane. A "fatal pathology" makes further repair pointless and painful. Some organ system, vital to life, is sputtering and about to quit. It may be the lungs, or the kidneys, or the digestive system. The sickness—not the doctor—has picked this organ system and is gradually sucking life out of the body.

While a good doctor or hospice care worker will try to land the plane gently and declare that repair work is pointless, a Dr. Kevorkian will say, "Look at that suffering airplane. Let's launch a surface-to-air missile to blow it out of the sky and put it out of its misery."

Do you see the difference? One strategy allows the natural dying process to take its course (the plane stops flying after its own internal problems—fatal pathology, if you will—have forced it to quit) while the other kills artificially and prematurely (a missile aborts the flight in mid-air by introducing its own fatal pathology).

I Don't Want to Endure Terrible Physical Suffering

Many cancer patients and their families, particularly in cancer's early stages, anticipate the future with fear because of the terrible physical pain they think is inevitable. This fear, however, is largely unfounded. Almost always, there is a way to greatly reduce or eliminate pain. Because some medications may impair clarity of thought, patients may prefer to endure a modicum of pain, however, in order to keep their minds clear. Sometimes, in the case of severe pain, patients may prefer to lapse into a state of deep sleep. But the use of pain medication is up to the patients. They and their loved ones should never feel guilty about using enough to eliminate pain.

At times the attempt to eliminate pain may hasten the dying process. But in a situation where the dying process has begun, there is nothing ethically wrong with such a choice. Nearly all ethicists agree that it is permissible to increase medication to control pain, even if premature death is a likely consequence. This is what ethicists call the double effect—the principle that allows an act to result in good and bad effects. Here, giving pain medication would have the primary intent (and effect) of relieving pain and the secondary effect of hastening death. Death is not the primary intent, as it is for Dr. Kevorkian.[6]

It should be clear, then, that the argument supporting physician-assisted suicide on the grounds of physical pain and unbearable suffering is rooted in ignorance and fear. Pain can be treated and symptoms controlled. Most cancer patients don't want to die early.

If there is a line of people at the door of state legislatures asking for legalization so that they can kill themselves, most are not cancer patients. A recent study at Boston's Dana-Farber Cancer Institute revealed that terminally ill cancer patients generally desired not death but pain relief. Patients experiencing unremitting pain were less interested in euthanasia or suicide than were the rest of the general public. Only those already in depression were interested in dying. In fact, this study found that patients who had once supported physician-assisted suicide changed their minds after they suffered with cancer: "There are big differences between what people say when they are talking theoretically and what they say when they are in real pain," said Dr. Ezekiel Emanuel, lead author of the Dana-Farber study. "Dying patients don't want to talk about death. They are often afraid that if they do, someone will offer to help them die."[7] Other studies have shown that physician-assisted suicide is virtually irrelevant when patients have high self-esteem, a sense of purpose, and friends.[8]

The physical suffering argument is a red herring for another reason. It is mental anguish not physical pain that supporters of suicide often most fear. They are afraid of losing beauty, function, or the freedom to enjoy their hobbies. A recent Dutch report showed that patients who requested euthanasia were concerned more with psychological than physical distress.[9] So the argument for physician-assisted suicide based on unrelenting pain is doubly wrong: Pain can be controlled, and euthanasia advocates most fear emotional distress.

What's more, psychological pain is often symptomatic of deeper, spiritual pain. In other words, even if the case for physical suffering had some merit, physician-assisted suicide would be problematic for a more important reason: It interferes with the process of spiritual healing. For non-Christians and Christians alike, there is often a burden of guilt that must be dealt with in the weeks or months before death. The awareness that death is approaching can be a healthy reminder from God that we must forgive and be forgiven to restore broken relationships. It is not enough, at these times, to simply be told that God forgives us. If we have sinned against another human being, we need to confess our sins to those we have sinned against and ask their forgiveness. Suicide often comes before patients have a chance to mend the fences that have been broken.

More than several of our patients have experienced the joy of reconciliation with estranged family and friends on their deathbeds. It is often painful, but the tears of joy that come with forgiveness are a priceless reward. They make dying so much easier.

I (Gerry) remember my aunt Helen who died more than thirty years ago as a thirty-four-year-old mother of three children. She had grown up in a religious home and had gone to church regularly, but still felt something was missing. It wasn't until cancer brought her to the portals of death, and she had a chance to ask questions of her sister Joan (my mother), who had recently come into a close relationship with Jesus, that Helen felt fully forgiven for her sins. She wept tears of joy, and told Joan that this was the happiest time of her life. Shortly after, she died—a happy and peaceful woman.

George was a sixty-year-old man in our church who died after a bout with kidney cancer. He had become a Christian shortly before doctors discovered his cancer. George survived nine months. During those months he had many uncomfortable moments, but he used the time to say good-bye to his children and, in one poignant moment, to be reconciled to one of them.

Neither Helen nor George would have enjoyed spiritual healing if they had committed suicide early in the process. Both died peaceful and happy deaths—far more peaceful and happy than they would have, had they allowed a physician to kill them before the natural cycle had been completed.

People usually kill themselves to avoid the rigors of the dying process. This is a principal reason why our society is beginning to embrace physician-assisted suicide: It is a convenient way to avoid the unpleasantness.

Death is now our strongest taboo. We don't want to talk about it (she "passed away," we say) and we certainly don't want to be reminded of its ultimate implications. So we either avoid the subject altogether, or we trivialize it, treating it as a natural process that shows how similar we are to animals and plants.

But this is an illusion. Death is indeed frightening. It separates us from those dear to us, disrupts our love relationships, and brings us face to face with God (a terrifying experience for those who do not know him but a wonderful one for those who do). This is why the saints of church history have always said that the unremitting remembrance of death is good for the soul. It induces the soul to prepare to meet its Creator. And it helps the soul to realize that the only solution to the horrors of death is the cross of Jesus Christ. Only his death can free us from the burden of our sinful guilt, and his resurrection gives us the brightest hope for life beyond death. Part of the evil of suicide is that it cuts the soul off prematurely from facing death and what it means. The soul is then less likely to recognize Jesus' salvation from eternal death.

For those who don't know Jesus, suicide is attractive because there appears to be little or no meaning to suffering. For many (but certainly not all) proponents of physician-assisted suicide, life is meaningless, "the tale told by an idiot, full of sound and fury, signifying nothing." As the bumper sticker puts it, "Life's a bitch and then you die." Since all is ultimately absurd, it is logical to make a quick exit before the going becomes too unpleasant. The answer to suffering, they reason, is to kill the sufferer. Suicide seems to be the answer to the pain of life. After all, they think, we have a right not to suffer.

For the Christian, however, suffering has meaning. It can be redemptive. As we have seen in previous chapters, it is not the ulti-mate evil. It can make us better people, and is part of what God arranges in our lives to bring us closer to himself. As Christian ethicist Stanley Hauerwas put it, "We rightly try to avoid unnecessary suffer-ing, but it also seems that we are never quite what we should be until we recognize the necessity and inevitability of suffering in our lives."[10]

Scripture tells us that suffering helps us share God's holiness, manifest the fruits of righteousness,[11] and grow in endurance, character, and hope.[12] Opting for suicide before our time has come can forestall this work of sanctification that God wants to perform in us.

It Puts Me in Charge of My Life

Proponents of physician-assisted suicide also argue that the option increases the freedom and autonomy of the patient. This is important, they say, because cancer limits their freedom, sometimes severely.

I could argue that insisting on freedom of choice buys into the value system of this fallen world, and that the Christian faith shows us that true freedom comes from submission to God's will. But for the sake of argument I will accept the premise that freedom to choose is always a good thing simply to show that in reality this "freedom" to kill themselves limits cancer patients' freedom in other important ways.

First, it breaks down trust in the doctor-patient relationship. If my doctor accepts the legitimacy of suicide and euthanasia, how can I be sure that my doctor will always try to heal me? And if my finances are unreliable, perhaps the doctor is shrewd enough to figure that I may not be able to pay the bills for long-term care. Now, the vast majority of oncologists would repudiate such mercenary thinking, so this may be farfetched. But in the Dana-Farber study cited earlier, most cancer patients felt they could not trust doctors who initiated discussions of physician-assisted suicide.

Second, it opens the door to abuse. If doctors know we are open to the possibility of suicide, they may be more likely to exploit this knowledge, albeit with good intentions. In the Netherlands, where physician-assisted suicide and euthanasia have been legalized, doctors have reported that they have given lethal injections to patients without those patients' formal approval.[13] There are also reports of newborns and infants being involuntarily euthanized in the Netherlands.[14] In fact, Dutch doctors reported in 1991 that they were doing two and one-half times more involuntary than voluntary physician-assisted suicides.[15]

Legalized physician-assisted suicide grants enormous power to physicians: They become judge, jury, and executioner. In the 1996 science fiction movie *Judge Dredd*, law and order in a futuristic city is ensured by street judges who ride the road, heavily armed, watching for people who break the law. When they see what they think is an offense, they summarily declare guilt, pass a sentence, and mete out justice right on the sidewalk. In one scene, Judge Dredd (Sylvester Stallone) discovers that a man has double-parked his car for the second time. The judge decides that this man needs to learn his lesson, so he demolishes the car.

This judicial overkill illustrates the danger of physician-assisted suicide. It invests physicians, like the street judges of the movie, with too much authority. They are empowered to diagnose "terminal illness," determine "competence," deliver the death sentence, and carry it out. With so much unchecked power, the risk of abuse is enormous.

Doctors are notorious for underrating patients' assessments of the quality of their lives because physicians often place too much emphasis on physical limitations and undervalue other capacities. They can also be surprised by unexpected recoveries. One of Bill's patients, Keith, tells the story of his mother who had breast cancer. Over a period of ten years, she had both breasts removed, along with the lymph nodes and muscles under her arms. Despite this treatment and chemotherapy, the cancer spread to her bones. She had more chemotherapy and then started sinking fast. When Keith reached her in the hospital, she was in a semiconscious state. Her doctors said there was nothing more they could do for her and asked Keith if they could disconnect all the tubes and just keep his mother as comfortable as possible. Keith granted permission. His mother was taken to a separate room to die comfortably.

To everyone's amazement, the next morning Keith's mother awoke, asked for something to eat, and checked herself out of the hospital at noon. She lived for another year and a half. My point is that doctors can be as surprised as anyone else (and sometimes more surprised) by a patient's unexpected recovery. Giving them unlimited power to decide when to kill a patient may rob that patient of more good months (perhaps years) of life.

This danger of unchecked power is usually ignored when the media discusses the right to die. Also ignored is the subtle loss of freedom that is disguised by the clamor to have a right to choose. That is, the move to maximize freedom makes the weak and elderly more vulnerable. The decision to increase options can actually reduce options. Allen Verhey has used the illustration of being invited to a party by a boor. "By increasing my options he effectively eliminated an option I suddenly realized I had the moment before but have no longer, the option I would have preferred—namely the option of both not spending three hours with this person and not explaining to him why I would rather not (or lying). The invitation increases my options, to be sure, but it also eliminates an option."[16]

Similarly, Verhey has argued, providing social and legal legitimation for assisted suicide eliminates the option of staying alive without having to justify one's existence. The burden will be hard to bear for someone who doesn't want to be a burden. Verhey reminds us of the practice of dueling, which gained its life from society's obsession with honor in the last century and before. Because dueling was an accepted method of resolving a dispute, it was very difficult to refuse a challenge to duel. We can only imagine how many men died because they didn't want, or didn't know how, to justify their desire not to duel.

As our society begins to accept and legitimize assisted suicide for cancer patients and others, it will be difficult for the weak to justify their existence to doctors and family who, for financial and other reasons, place subtle pressure on patients not to be a "burden" any longer. It will be especially difficult when doctors and third-party payers are concerned about saving valuable resources, and may cause some physicians to ignore other methods of relieving pain and suffering. Those patients who will feel the pressure the most will be the elderly and socially nonproductive. The strong will use this pressure to get rid of the weak.

So increasing our freedom of choice actually limits our freedom both by breaking down trust in the patient-doctor relationship and opening the door to abuse. There's a third way that we are limited by this freedom: it corrupts us. To the extent that we condone and participate in killing those who are not actually dying, we will be tainted by what Pope John Paul II has called the "culture of death." Just as soldiers returning from battle feel coarsened by the killing they have seen and done, we will be debased by the killing we have aided or abetted. Aristotle said that an act contributes to a habit, which shapes a character, which then becomes a destiny. If we participate in assisted suicide, we help form a habit and character at odds with God's kingdom of life. We will then be less free to see and enjoy the "glorious liberty of the children of God."[17] For we shall have usurped God's prerogative of deciding who will live and when to die. This is to make an idol of the self, which, when hardened by habit, is difficult to destroy. Once they are on the throne, rulers are loath to get off.

Life Is Not Worth Living without a Minimum of Quality

The quality of life argument takes two forms today. On the one hand, there are cancer (and other) patients who say they don't want to endure life once they have lost a certain level of function or enjoyment. Then there are those—doctors, hospital administrators, and public policy experts who are concerned about limited resources and escalating costs, and anticipate the rationing of medical care—who say that some lives are worth less than others. These latter folks tend to reduce individuals to statistical profiles: "She's eighty years old. There's no sense keeping her alive any longer. People that age need to give way to those who are still making a contribution." Sanctity of life has been replaced by quality of life.

The problem with both of these attitudes is that they presume we can know the value of a person's life—either our own or someone else's. There is not a shred of biblical support for this presumption. Quite the contrary: The Scriptures tell us that all human beings are made in God's image,[18] so an individual's worth is connected to God's very being. It is conferred by God, not society. Society tends to diminish the value of the weak and vulnerable, but Jesus identified himself with these: "I was hungry . . . I was thirsty . . . I was a stranger . . . naked

. . . sick and in prison . . . as you [helped those in these conditions], you did it to me."[19] We may wonder how a very old person or deformed infant could have value, but their worth, as the Swiss theologian Karl Barth put it, is "God's little secret."

How many of us realize that the quality of life argument is directly at odds with the Declaration of Independence? In that document, which is universally recognized as a foundation for the American experiment, Thomas Jefferson declared that "all men are created equal, endowed by their Creator with inalienable rights: life, liberty and the pursuit of happiness." If all human beings are equal, it makes no sense to say that some lives are more valuable than others. That would be to say that some are more equal than others!

The Slippery Slope

The quality of life approach to sickness, both for cancer and other diseases, is dangerous because of what it may encourage. Former Surgeon General C. Everett Koop believes that widespread acceptance of this premise will reduce the commitment of health care professionals to saving human life:

> If [we allow the] Downs syndrome or spina bifida [baby to die], what about AIDS or the crack baby? If one set of patients can be eliminated at will, the whole spirit of struggling to save lives is lost. Before long, a doctor or nurse [will think], "Why try so hard on anyone? After all, we deliberately fail to treat some and kill others. If the mongoloid is fair game, what about the blind and deaf? If the hopeless cripple confined to a wheelchair, what about the frail, retarded, senile? Cystic fibrosis, diabetes? The obese person who needs an inordinate amount of food to sustain his body?"[20]

Accepting the quality of life premise has implications for our whole society. It was just this assumption—that some lives are more valuable than others—that allowed Germans in the thirties to kill certain citizens. Physician and novelist Walker Percy has pointed out that the most influential German book in the 1920s was *The Justification of the*

Destruction of Life Devoid of Value, written by the distinguished jurist Karl Binding and the noted psychiatrist Alfred Hoche.[21] Robert Lifton, author of *The Nazi Doctors*, argued that the Nazi genocide started from small beginnings—a subtle shift in thinking that permitted people to believe there are lives not worthy to be lived.[22] Percy recently suggested that the quality of life argument, typically made in the name of compassion, leads inevitably to "the gas chamber," societies where "mercy killings" are used for not only the terminally ill but also those deemed socially useless.[23]

Other Christian Arguments against Assisted Suicide

So far our arguments against assisted suicide have mostly used reasons accessible to Christians and non-Christians alike. Before I close this chapter, let's look more explicitly at Christian reasons for opposing suicide.

First, suicide is a sin against faith. German theologian Dietrich Bonhoeffer (who was martyred by the Nazis) characterized suicide as a lack of faith in God's wisdom. God has reserved for himself the right to determine the end of life because he alone knows the goal to which it is his will to lead it. If we take our lives in our own time, we fail to trust God's wisdom in ending life in his time.

Nowhere does the Bible expressly forbid suicide, but the suicides that are mentioned are usually the result of extremely grave sin—by, for example, the traitor Ahithophel (who betrayed David) and Judas. While suicide is treated as a serious sin, it is not the unforgivable sin. Only rejecting Jesus and the Gospel, after they have been presented and understood, is unforgivable. This is clear from the context of Jesus' remarks about the unforgivable sin: he was responding to the Pharisees' declaration that he was an agent of Satan, thus rejecting his claim that he came from God.[24] It is this denial of Jesus' claim to be who he said he was (not suicide) that is the unforgivable sin against the Holy Spirit. Just as there will be murderers such as David, in heaven, so too there will be suicides enjoying eternal life with God and the other saints.

Suicide is a sin against faith in God's providence. Most suicides believe their lives serve no good purpose. But the Book of Job reveals that our lives can serve a purpose that is completely hidden to us. The author of Job told his readers that Job's terrible trials were for the purpose of demonstrating faithfulness to the spiritual world. This purpose was never revealed to Job, but he nevertheless refused his wife's advice to commit suicide.[25] Although he spent more than thirty chapters shaking his fist in anger and bitterness toward God, he never gave up on God (see our discussion of Job in chapter 12).

Similarly, suicide is a sin against faith in God's sovereignty. Some suicides presuppose that we own our own lives, and therefore can control them. But, as Bertrand Russell famously said, "Presupposition has all the advantages over demonstration that theft has over honest labor." The reality is that God owns us. He created every speck of our protoplasm, and we continue to exist moment to moment only because his Son continues to uphold us.[26] As the psalmist wrote, "The Lord is God. It is he that made us, and we are his."[27]

Second, suicide is a sin against the sixth commandment ("You shall not murder"), particularly because it is often undertaken without consideration of the needs and hopes of others. The church fathers said that relinquishing one's life is permissible if it is for the purpose of serving others—in the performance of duty in military service, in the defense of a friend unjustly attacked, in ministering to infectious sick, in witnessing to faith in persecution. But these cases are different from suicide, which is committed for selfish reasons, such as wounded honor, erotic passion, financial ruin, gambling debts, or shame over serious personal lapses.

When I was principal of a private school in Minnesota, a young father of three young children made some bad investments and wound up in deep debt. In a fit of panic, he killed himself. His wife and children were traumatized; they felt abandoned by a man who had pledged to care for them and were thrown into a financial tailspin from which it took years to recover. I'm not sure that his children will ever fully recover emotionally.

Third, suicide is a violation of Jesus' command to love. It prematurely deprives the family and community of a valuable person, and denies others the opportunity of ministering to that person's needs.

A neighbor of mine lost her cancer-stricken father to suicide because he was afraid he wouldn't be able to pay his hospital bills. This was an irrational fear because he had adequate insurance. My neighbor mourns the loss of the many months, perhaps even years, she could have had with her father. (And what about the loss of hope of recovery? Many with terminal illnesses, including cancer, can live for years and lead meaningful, happy lives during that time.)

A Middle Way

In a society that increasingly embraces a culture of death, rejection of assisted suicide may come to be seen as an extremist position. But it is really a middle way between two dangerously extreme views. One extreme demands all possible medical treatment for any serious condition and refuses to ever let the patient die—either because unbelievers see this life as our only hope, or because believers have the misguided view that God always wants to heal every physical illness. The other extreme wants to eliminate suffering altogether and so insists on both active euthanasia and the right to physician-assisted suicide.

Both positions are idolatrous. That is, both make an idol of the human self—either in its earthly life or in its power to control God. One says that human existence on earth is ultimate or that human beings can control God by their faith, while the other takes God's place of determining who is worthy of life and when it should end. Neither trusts God's wisdom and love to order our lives.

15

What Is Hospice?

Dying with Dignity

L ittle more than a week earlier Gloria had thought she had been in
perfect health. At seventy-two, she could easily pass for sixty-two,
and had felt fine for years. Gloria had always thought that if she died
from a disease, it would be lung cancer, since she was a heavy smoker.

That Sunday Gloria's husband, Tom, woke up to find her twitching
in bed. She was in the midst of a seizure. After he got her to the hospital and doctors had run their tests on her, he was shocked to hear she
had a brain tumor. Specialists told him it could be traced to a large
kidney cancer that had spread to the liver, bones, and then brain.

I (Bill) saw both Gloria and Tom in my office. It was a difficult visit.
Just a few days before, life had seemed glorious, with prospects for a
long and happy future; but now, after what seemed only a few hours,
doctors told them that Gloria had very little time to live.

Gloria is a tall, attractive accountant, who speaks with a husky
voice. Tom is a thin, fit electrical engineer—quiet and kind. Both
were strangely calm as I told them about the several treatment options

available to them and that there was only a 10 to 20 percent chance that any of them would increase the quality or quantity of Gloria's life. None offered any hope of cure.

Gloria replied firmly, "I don't want to subject myself or my family to those treatments. A twenty percent chance isn't good enough. If this is my time to go, let's just get on with it."

Tom was half-crying and half-smiling as he listened to his wife explain that she wanted to be in control of her dying; she refused to be strapped to tubes that delivered drugs that might not help her and could even make her feel worse.

It was at that point that I told her about the hospice alternative. She could die at home, with a minimum of discomfort, and in the midst of her family. I explained that it would mean giving up medical attempts to make her life longer and that in many cases as a result it makes life better. And by making life better, it might offer a longer—perhaps even much longer—life.

"That's what I want!" Gloria exclaimed. Tom smiled and squeezed her hand while she continued. "I want my family to be around, without having to go to the hospital. I want them to be able to change my sheets, and feed me, and take me to the store, and talk with me until the end. This is the gift I want to give them. That is how I want to be remembered—not to die alone, in the hospital, with some stranger calling them in the middle of the night telling them I'm gone."

"I think you'll like the way the hospice folks care for you," I assured Gloria. "The hospice nurse will be almost like family to you. She'll know the floorplan of your house, the driveway, even where the dog's chain ends. Since you live out in the country, she and others will get reflector tape and put it on the trees and fenceposts at turns on the way out to your house so hospice workers don't get lost. 'Follow the blue tapes,' they'll tell one another.

"And you won't have to worry about pain and other discomforts. They may not all be eliminated, but you can always call the nurse whenever you need help with them, and he or she will do whatever can be done to minimize them. The nurse will give you the same pain medicines you would get in the hospital.

"You'll also find, Gloria, that this is a great time to build bridges and mend fences. You can heal any relationships that need healing and close your life with renewed love for your family and friends."

Gloria and Tom left my office looking like they'd just been told that she was cured. They were positively beaming! (You may not believe me if you have never seen hospice at work. Please read on.)

Hospice (in most communities) means dying at home. It is dying, but with good control of pain and discomfort, and with a sense of peace because there has been spiritual preparation for death. Most important, the patient is surrounded with family and friends.

A Little History

The idea has been around for centuries, but it was only a few decades ago that an organization was started to help people put the idea into practice. In 1967 Dame Cicely Saunders opened St. Christopher's Hospice in Sydenham (a district of London), England, with the intent of offering a comprehensive approach to care for the dying. Dame Saunders insisted that the dying always get the best relief possible of physical suffering and that attention also be given to the social, psychological, and spiritual factors affecting the patient and family. Ten years later her idea caught on across the Atlantic; hospices in the United States have been springing up ever since. At this writing there are more than 2,000 hospices in America.

I was very skeptical about hospices when I first started to look into them seven years ago. I thought they offered little more than hand holding. I was convinced—naively and perhaps arrogantly—that no one could care for the dying as well as I could. And I worried that if I got involved (the folks at Good Samaritan Hospice in Roanoke had invited me to be their medical director), I would be faced with another blizzard of paperwork, intended to make my life miserable.

Getting the Facts

But I discovered I was wrong on this and almost all my other preconceptions about hospice. Soon I got the facts:

- Hospice care is intended for patients who no longer have any realistic hope for cure and choose to remain at home.

- A life expectancy of six months or less is the basic criterion for enrollment. However, some stay for up to several years.

- Malignant diseases account for the majority of hospice entries, but others include heart disease, lung disease, and AIDS.

- A hospice is usually not a place but a team of caregivers.

- When you enter hospice, you agree to give up chemotherapy, radiation, and most forms of artificial life support (except in extreme circumstances).

- Most insurers, including Medicare and Medicaid, will pay for hospice.

Benefits

I also learned that the list of hospice benefits is long. For the sake of easy viewing, I will list them and describe each briefly.

Team Caring

Perhaps the greatest benefit is the team of professionals (doctors, nurses, social service workers) who come to care for you and love you as you go through the end of your life. At Good Samaritan Hospice, our team meetings begin and end with prayer. In between are tears, laughter, and concerns shared by each professional. We care not just for the patient but for the entire circle of loved ones. When the patient is alone, we make sure caring takes place at a nursing home or someone else's home—unless the patient is still self-sufficient. The important thing is that when you are in hospice, you have a team of trained people dedicated to making this critical process as comfortable as possible.

The Art of Pain Management

One of the biggest reasons for the growing interest in Dr. Kevorkian's approach to dying is fear of pain. I am convinced that far fewer cancer patients would consider the Kevorkian plan if they knew that at hospices pain management has been elevated to an art form. The entire team works diligently to eliminate or minimize pain. Cancer pain control is the foundation upon which hospice care rests.

But it is not just pain that hospice workers labor to relieve. They also work to maintain good hygiene and reduce anxiety, sleeplessness, shortness of breath, constipation, and skin breakdown.

There are other symptoms that hospice workers are not as concerned about because they are natural signs of impending death: weight loss, poor appetite, weakness, and decreasing levels of awareness. We may not want to see or hear about these symptoms, but they are natural at the end of life. They are difficult to treat, and what's more, don't need to be treated.

Help with Messy Details

When someone is dying, it is difficult to keep up with all the bureaucratic details that sometimes come in torrents. This is where the hospice social worker comes in. This person carries the huge burden of coordinating benefits, arranging home health equipment, and trouble-shooting special problem areas within the family that need to be addressed.

The Personal Touch

Then there's the home health aid. This person is more "hands-on" than anyone else on the team. She or he will help the patient stay clean and bathed. Some of the closest bonding I have seen has been between these home health aids and the families they have helped. Beautiful relationships of love have formed.

Counseling and Spiritual Support

Cancer patients who are dying often have questions about the dying process, death, God, and life after death that demand answers. Many of the questions we dealt with in chapters 9 through 13 are asked over and over again in hospice—such as Why me, God? Is cancer part of God's plan? What if there is no reason? and How can I cope?

Thankfully, here it is not wrong to ask these kinds of questions, and many hospice personnel are prepared to help patients work through them. The aim of their counseling, however, is not necessarily to provide sure-fire answers, but to listen patiently and empathetically, or point patients to Scripture and inspirational reading. Often the best comfort they give is simply to provide a shoulder to cry on.

In times like these, hospice workers often are privileged to see scenes of great love and beauty. Not long ago, we took care of Dana, a young mother whose courage was a shining beam of light to her husband, three young children, and all of us on the hospice team throughout her year-long battle with breast cancer. One of Dana's goals was to see Matthew, her five-year-old son, get on the school bus and begin kindergarten. By the grace of God and true grit, she achieved her goal. In September of that year, with tears running down her cheeks, she smiled with joy from her bedroom window as she watched Matthew board the school bus and turn around and wave from the top step.

Part of Matthew's new kindergarten experience was to begin a Christmas fund at the suggestion of his teacher. Each child was supposed to contribute a nickel or dime each week; in December, the students would each buy a Christmas present for one of their parents, wrap it, and place it under the classroom tree.

As Dana's cancer progressed, it became clear that she would not make it to Christmas Day. At the same time she knew that the gift her son had purchased was a tiny imitation diamond ring. Because she knew that her time was short, she started to ask Matthew if she could open her present.

Matthew was adamant in his refusal. "Mom, you always tell me not to open my presents early. So you shouldn't either!"

Dana knew she couldn't open it without confusing her little boy. So she promised him she'd wait till Christmas Day. Unfortunately, she didn't live that long. The Lord took her home two weeks before Christmas—at home, surrounded by loved ones.

At the funeral, those of us who knew about the ring were overwhelmed when we saw on Dana's ring finger—in place of her wedding ring—a tiny imitation diamond ring. Little Matthew had put it on his mother's finger. We heard later that just before she died, Dana had instructed her husband to give Matthew her wedding ring as a memory of her love for him, and to tell their little boy that his mom would be proud to wear his ring to heaven.

Sometimes hospice workers are asked if they don't get depressed by all the dying they see. It is moments like these that make us want to keep coming back. It's at hospice that we are given the gift of seeing the meaning of life while caring for those tasting death.

A Better Life

Some patients have trouble giving up their hope of a cure when they enter hospice. I try to reassure them that while entering hospice is a step back from the medical model of cure, it is a step forward in living out the rest of their lives. In fact, I explain, life in hospice is not only better but also often longer for a number of reasons. Pain is usually better controlled than in the hospital, and potentially toxic tests and therapies are stopped. Besides, once you are at home, out of pain, and not making regular visits to the doctor, life often looks a little better.

One of our first hospice patients was an energetic, self-made entrepreneur named Ned, who looked at his incurable pancreas cancer as yet another challenge in life. He had conquered so many obstacles before, and this seemed like another great adventure.

Ned made lists of things he wanted to do, people he wanted to see and meet, old enemies he needed to be reconciled with, and even a few more business transactions he wanted to conduct. Throwing himself into these projects with gusto, he also made sure his wife had every possible financial security, rewrote his will, prepared a living will (see chapter 16), and visited a host of friends (and former adversaries!).

Once he completed his list of things to do, Ned sat and waited for the end to come. And waited. And waited. Since his pancreas cancer was not fast growing, his pain was so well controlled, and he could eat and drink and get around in his car, the dying process was not coming fast enough for him! Soon our hospice team was having trouble finding him when it came out to make rounds.

Of course Ned eventually succumbed to cancer. But the end of his life illustrated so much of what is good about hospice. Ned's symptoms were controlled, he made his own decisions about the end of his life and carried them out, and he healed a number of wounds in relationships that were still festering when he discovered he had terminal cancer. Ned left this earth not by his own hand, but in his own due time and at peace.

It's Less Expensive!

Another advantage of hospice is that it greatly reduces the financial strain on both patients and their families because it usually saves money. This is primarily because of the Medicare hospice benefit. You may recall from chapter 7 that Medicare is divided between Part A and Part B. When Medicare patients enroll in hospice, they give up traditional care (chemo, radiation, and hospital treatment) provided under Part A but continue to receive all the benefits of Part B.

Now the good news may be hard to believe. While traditional (hospital) treatment under Medicare has copayments, deductibles, and only 80 percent coverage for most services, almost all hospice services are 100 percent paid for by Medicare! This is truly a breakthrough in caring for people at what may be the most trying time of their lives. Patients and their families can derive comfort from knowing that at least this stage of their illness will not hurt them financially.

What hospice services are provided for by Medicare? The list includes nearly everything needed:

- Doctor's care

- Registered nurse visits

- Medical appliances and supplies

- Prescription medications for pain relief and symptom management

- Short-term hospital care if needed, including respite care (rare occasions when a caregiver—usually a spouse—has an over-whelming need for a break; the patient goes to the hospital for a few days while the caregiver gets a much-needed rest)

- Home health aid (see The Personal Touch above)

- Physical therapy, occupational therapy, speech and language pathology services (for patients who have lost use of their voice box)

- Medical social service (see Help with Messy Details above)

- Counseling and spiritual support

I must add that even if you don't qualify for Medicare, your insurance probably covers most of these hospice services.

Restrictions

If you are considering hospice, you also need to know there are four benefit periods in hospice. These are to prevent the system from being abused. The first two benefit periods are each ninety days long (for a total of six months). The third period is thirty days, during which time it is determined whether the patient is truly dying, as originally thought, or if it has become clear that she or he will live many more months (or even years). If the patient then enters the fourth benefit period, which is indefinite, and at some point leaves hospice because she or he is doing so well, the patient will not be permitted to return.

This may strike you as odd, but it helps protect Medicare and hospices from fraud. If these restrictions did not exist, patients could go into hospice, then go to a hospital to receive more expensive traditional medical care, and return to hospice—and continue this cycle indefinitely while costing both systems multiplied thousands of dollars. The hospice benefit is intended to assist patients in their dying months, not milk the system for as much insurance benefit as possible.

Dying Well

There is one last benefit that is not always mentioned in discussions of the hospice alternative. It teaches the survivors how to die well. Not knowing how to die well is one result of our society's fixation on medical cure and fear of facing death. This is why Dr. Kevorkian's approach is attractive to so many. But it is also why hospice is so desperately needed. It teaches beautiful lessons to all those involved that there are better things than taking the quickest possible exit when death approaches. It shows the rest of us how to die with true dignity.

16

Is There
Life after Cancer?

---

*How to Live Day to Day
Once Everything Has Changed*

At sixty-two, Roger had experienced the ups and downs of an exciting life. He had owned successful businesses in New York and a gold mine in Colorado. He had married and fathered three healthy children. But then the business climate soured; he lost most of his money and his marriage as well. He became estranged from his children. And to top it all, he discovered he had inoperable cancer. His doctor said he would be surprised if Roger lived much beyond two weeks.

Cancer forced Roger to look hard at his life, and some remarkable changes resulted. The Christian faith that he had discovered shortly before his cancer diagnosis came alive with a new power. He pushed himself to seek out his children, two of whom lived hundreds of miles away. Old wounds were healed, and new love blossomed. The new Roger found a special delight in showing care for people: He hugged and prayed for people who were hurting, went out of his way to get a tape player for a friend's speech therapy, and brought pizza unannounced to a Bible study group in his church. When Roger died, eight months after his diagnosis, he died at peace with God, himself, and others.

Linnea was deeply shocked to learn that the little lump under her arm was a malignant tumor. Almost before she could process what was happening to her, she was in the hospital, recovering from a mastectomy. Then, a few days after her operation, she woke up to realize that, even though all signs of her cancer were gone, life would never be the same for her. She was right. It has now been ten years since her operation, and her life since that time has been different indeed.

Outwardly, Linnea's patterns have not changed remarkably. She is still a busy homemaker, very active in the lives of her husband, children, friends, and church and community groups. But her outlook has changed. Now she is careful not to abuse her body. She tries to eat nutritious, low-fat foods, and she jogs with a friend five days a week. She lives one day at a time, savoring the little blessings of life. "Now I take time to smell the flowers," she says. "My brush with death made me realize that I was rushing too fast through life, that I wasn't taking enough time to enjoy people or to appreciate the little gifts that every day brings."

The View from the Edge of the Cliff

Linnea survived cancer, and Roger didn't. But both were able to use cancer to become better human beings. Both conquered cancer by allowing cancer to teach them how to live differently. Can you do the same? We believe that you can. But first you must face up to something few of us like to acknowledge.

There are two worlds in human existence. One is earthly life, the one we inhabit every day. The other is the world of the afterlife, when our present physical body ceases to exist.

Every one of us, in other words, will one day die and face the next world. But some of us don't want to think about our own deaths. Perhaps we find it too frightening. Or we feel guilty because we know what we haven't done in life. Some are simply convinced there is no life after death. So they go through their days with both feet planted firmly on this earth, letting days go by with little thought of death and the possibility of life beyond.

They are poorer as a result. Not financially poorer, of course, but poorer spiritually. It has been the testimony of countless generations that those who squarely face the certainty of their deaths enjoy a richer and more meaningful life. Those who summon the courage to contemplate their mortality tend to be more focused on the important things of life, less apt to be driven to pursuits that they will regret in the long run.

Few things carry us to the border zone between these two worlds more quickly than a diagnosis of cancer, which pulls us up to this precipice and forces us to face the reality we so easily ignore—death. Some of us, like Roger, will pass over the precipice fairly quickly after the diagnosis of cancer. Others, like Linnea, will lean over the precipice and peer carefully at the other world, then move back (for a while) to a safety zone far from the border. They will have won the physical battle against cancer—yet their lives will be changed irrevocably.

Imagine, then, that you are standing on the edge of this cliff we have been describing and looking over to the other side. What do you still want to accomplish before you have to cross over? Whom do you need to love? Where do you need to go? How do you need to change your priorities? A good place to start is with your relationships.

The People in Your Life

Many people who discover they have cancer suddenly realize that they have not put the time and energy into their important relationships that they should have. They come to see that they have thought far more of themselves than they have of others, and that people are hurting as a result. Some realize they have concentrated so much on getting ahead in the world that they have virtually ignored the real needs of those around them.

If you have come to a similar realization, take this opportunity to focus on what you may have long put on a back burner: your relationships. No matter what your age, it is never too late to start showing love to others. Try to think of others' needs, not just your own.

Some of us—men, especially—have been raised to believe that it is not manly or proper to express our feelings to the people we care about, or that words are relatively unnecessary as long as we do our work to help provide. But people need words. They want to be talked to. They generally want to hear how we feel about things as well as how we think about things.

You may have some broken relationships, perhaps even with people in your own family. There may be some people you have decided never to speak to or see again. Perhaps they hurt you, and this is your way of paying them back. Or maybe there are people who have done this to you. In either case, a wall of hurt or anger or bitterness or indifference has grown up between you.

Wouldn't it be wonderful to restore these relationships in the months (or years) that are remaining to you? Wouldn't you like to know that you have done everything you could to do what's right in this world before you passed out of it? The good news is that you can. And there are two simple ways of doing this.

The first is to ask forgiveness of those you have wronged. Think about those broken relationships. Did you do something that might have offended or hurt the other person? Even if it was years ago, and even if you cannot possibly understand why your word or deed could have caused such offense, the fact remains that the other person was wounded by what you did. You should ask forgiveness for it.

Don't just say, "I'm sorry." The other person is probably sorry also. But the wall may remain between you if neither has acknowledged wrongdoing. Take the initiative by saying, "I was wrong," even if you were responsible for only 5 percent of the problem. Those three words, "I was wrong," have a magical power to open the most hardened heart. Then ask the other person if he or she will forgive you.

It may not be easy, but it's not as hard as you think. If you are forgiven, you will feel the joy of a healed relationship. The burden of guilt will lift from your shoulders. Even if the other person does not forgive you, you will have the peace and self-respect that come from knowing that you have done everything you could to make things right.

The other key is to forgive those who have hurt or offended you. Punishing people by holding a grudge may provide some satisfaction, but forgiveness gives far more. Better yet, forgiveness frees us from the terrible burden of bitterness and resentment.

Years ago, I (Gerry) was demoted in a job by people I had considered friends. To my mind, their reasons for demoting me were unfounded. Their implicit lack of confidence in me was, I thought, unjustified. For days I stewed with anger and resentment. I could not look these people in the eye. I felt hatred for people I had once cared about.

Finally, however, I realized that bitterness was hurting me spiritually and emotionally and was even making me physically sick. So I decided to confront the people involved, tell them what I thought as politely and calmly as I could, and then forgive them. I did so two days later. As soon as I walked out of the meeting, I felt freed from an enormous weight. They did not change their decision, but I had gotten my feelings off my chest and had made the decision to forgive. I could smile again.

Sometimes, of course, forgiveness does not come so easily and quickly; it may take months or even years. Cases of deep-seated hurt or bitterness may require repeated prayers for the willingness and power to forgive. But even if the feeling of resentment remains, you have still made a start, an effort to forgive. And regardless of how you feel, the attitude of your mind has already changed. You have already become a better human being. If you persist in your efforts, you will eventually be free of your bitterness.

The marvelous thing about asking for forgiveness and forgiving others is the richer life these changes in relationship can bring. If cancer brings us across the precipice, we can die in peace. If we survive cancer, we can go on to live a richer life of love. In either case, whether we die sooner or later, we have conquered cancer by using it to become better people.

Perhaps you are one of those who already concentrate more on people than things. You know that maintaining healthy and loving relationships takes work under the best of circumstances. Even then, you will probably find that cancer brings new stresses to your relationships: financial strain, changes in sexuality, mood swings, difficulties in communication.

Your marriage, for instance, may feel the strain, even if your relationship has been relatively harmonious. If your marriage has been rocky, cancer may make it even rockier. Our point is not to scare you, but to advise you that more care than normal is needed to protect your relationship under the tremendous stress of serious illness. It will be difficult to put extra effort into a relationship when you are being tossed by waves of fear, but a forewarning can prevent you from being blown overboard by a sudden gale. This is the time to take advantage of community agencies that provide help for troubled marriages. Check particularly for a local chapter of the American Cancer Society and their I Can Cope programs. These programs can help you understand the changes that cancer brings to a relationship and help you take positive steps to deal with them.

The Work You Have to Do

Not only marriage and relationships will be affected by cancer. Work and ordinary responsibilities around the home will change as well. Cancer patients will probably have more difficulty working on the job and at some points may be unable to go to work at all. And patients who are responsible for running a household may have enormous difficulty keeping up their usual pace.

In both cases, the burden of responsibility will have to shift to other members of the family. The patient's loved ones should expect to pick up more of the load. They will have to perform tasks that the cancer patient once took care of. This shift of workload may add stress to an atmosphere the cancer diagnosis has already strained.

The situation can become particularly difficult when the patient is a spouse who has taken care of the house and provided meals for her or his mate. The mate comes home to a house that was once immaculate, only to find that his or her work has just begun. And the sick spouse, who once was independent and in control of the home, may feel completely disoriented. For the first time the patient seems absolutely dependent on other people, and a once well-ordered home seems in shambles.

This is the bad news. The good news is that none of these problems is insurmountable. Many patients have survived—and learned from— far worse experiences and have overcome. The key is for cancer patients and their families to examine their expectations and to change them when necessary.

In other words, expect that less will be done in the same amount of time. Expect mood swings and sudden flare-ups of anger. Then compensate—first by focusing on what is most important, then by doing what is needed to maintain relationships and keep the home in reasonable order. Be prepared to let some things slide to avoid neglecting more important ones—light a candle to hide the dust and then snuggle to read to a child. And be prepared to go the extra mile for the patient who is having trouble walking at all.

If you mentally prepare yourself for these challenges and resolve to work through them, you can overcome. But you probably can't do it alone; you will probably need to ask for help. Don't be too bashful or too proud to ask for and accept help from relatives, from church, from the friends who say, "Call if you need anything."

It may be really hard to call a neighbor and say, "Well, the thing that would really help is if you could keep our lawn mowed for a while," or to call a friend with "Could you keep the kids today? My chemo has just wiped me out." But calling for help might be a life-saver—and the neighbor or friend will feel better for having done it. Keep in mind that many people don't help because they don't know what to do.

If you are a believer, this is the time to draw on your spiritual resources. Now, more than ever, is when you need God. Don't neglect personal prayer, time with your pastor, or friends from church. You may be tempted to forego these times and relationships if God seems distant, but they can give you the spiritual support you desperately need.

Above all, resolve to fight the temptation to give up, to walk away from it all by deserting your family or even committing suicide (see chapter 14). If you walk away, cancer has conquered you by destroying your spirit. Then cancer destroys not just one life, but many. The experience of thousands of cancer patients demonstrates that does not have to happen.

Your Self-Image: "What's Happened to Me?"

Some cancers (and their treatments) do little to alter a patient's physical appearance. But others bring drastic changes—and those changes can be traumatic. We all look at ourselves in the mirror and shower each day. What happens when the person we see is missing a body part—or an entire head of hair? How does the sudden gain—or loss—of thirty pounds affect the way we feel about ourselves?

Because our society attaches so much importance to physical appearance, we tend to think less of ourselves when these changes happen to us. We imagine that people will not like us as much or may even be repulsed by them. Some patients are afraid to go out in public for fear of what others will think. Many patients say they don't like themselves because of what has happened to their bodies.

It's important to realize that these feelings are natural. We were created with bodies, and at least in this life our bodies are inseparable from our persons. What happens to our bodies will always affect the way we feel about ourselves.

You may want to try one or more of these strategies when you are embarrassed by your body:

- Don't hesitate to do what you can to feel better about your appearance. Buy a wig or a prosthesis if that helps. Or visit a local salon for a makeover.

- Talk about your fears and embarrassment with trusted friends.

- Write out Scripture passages that remind you how precious you are to God (with or without a "normal" body)—for example, Psalms 139:13–16, Matthew 6:25–27, and Isaiah 43:1–5.

- Try helping others. Making a difference in someone else's life will help you feel better about yourself.

- Try a little humor. Tell a wig joke to a friend.

Finally, try not to forget (it is easy to forget because the media and much of the world tell us otherwise) that who we are is not determined by how we look, but by our inner character. What counts in the end is not what we look like, but how we treat people and how we respond to God.

What You Can Do—Practical Steps

Now that you have come up to the edge of the precipice, how do you change your living patterns? There are a number of practical steps you can take to live a new kind of life. We will focus on them in the next few pages, then outline some specific personal and spiritual strategies you should consider.

Rally Your Resources

The first practical step is to contact local and national resources to help you get through the difficult days ahead. You are not alone in your battle against cancer. Millions of patients have gone ahead of you. You may have a network of friends and family already in place. And a host of professional people and organizations—nurses, social workers, beauticians, members of the clergy, cancer societies, psychologists, nutritionists, and physical therapists—stand ready to help you. Here are some of the programs they have developed to provide that help (see the appendix for addresses, phone numbers, and other details):

- The American Cancer Society is a well-established, nonprofit organization with chapters in most communities. The Society promotes cancer education and prevention and provides support for cancer patients. This is a good place to learn more about your cancer and to find people with whom you can talk.

- The National Cancer Institute provides a Cancer Information Service that offers medical and technical information to help you understand and decide about treatment options and possibilities.

- Reach to Recovery is a group of volunteer women who have undergone mastectomy (removal of a breast) and are eager to provide support for women in the same situation. Call your local cancer society to get in touch with a local chapter of this group.

- The Look Good . . . Feel Better program is offered by the Cosmetic, Toiletry, and Fragrance Association Foundation in partnership with the American Cancer Society and the National Cosmetology Association. This is another free service that seeks to promote health by helping the cancer patient look as good as possible.

- I Can Cope is a series of meetings of varying length, usually free, put on by local chapters of the American Cancer Society. It gives you an opportunity to listen and respond to local cancer experts—doctors, nurses, technicians, psychiatrists, and clergy. The I Can Cope series is a good place to begin asking questions although it is not set up for one-on-one counseling. That is best left to the physician and pastor who are caring for the patient.

- Support groups are offered by many local cancer centers and hospitals, which sponsor both daytime and evening meetings where patients and their families can share stories and support one another. Cancer support groups arc usually directed by trained professionals who work with cancer patients or may have had cancer themselves.

  Support groups are not for everyone. You may feel you get enough support from family or friends, or you may prefer to deal with your concerns in the quiet of your innermost self. But if you feel better talking about your condition openly and would benefit from hearing from those who also have cancer, then a support group can be a source of great strength. It can give you an opportunity to share your feelings with those who understand.

- Ronald McDonald Houses are offered in many communities with major hospitals. These homes, sponsored by the McDonald's Corporation, give parents a place to stay while their seriously ill children are being treated. A very modest nightly payment is requested, but the charge is waived if the family cannot afford it. Ronald McDonald houses are located in more than 120 cities in the United States, Europe, Canada, and Australia.

- National Hospice Organization programs provide medical, spiritual, and psychological care to dying patients and their families, usually in the home (see chapter 15). They aim to enhance the quality of a terminal patient's remaining life by preventing unwanted testing and hospitalization, offering pain relief, and helping patients and families prepare for death.

Get Your Affairs in Order

Even though a diagnosis of cancer is far from the hopeless situation some people fear, it is still a serious and sometimes fatal disease. You can provide yourself and your family with peace of mind and cut down on your stress levels by taking care of some basic legal and financial matters as soon as possible.

Make a Will

Everyone should have a will, but it's especially important that a cancer patient have one. Your attorney can help you construct a legal document that states your wishes for what takes place after your death. Even if it is clear that you will survive your cancer, you owe it to your loved ones to make this provision. (After all, you could die in a car accident on the way to the hospital.) Without the protection of a will, a larger portion of your assets than you would want might go to the government.

If your estate is very simple, do-it-yourself will kits or computer programs could help you draw up a basic document that is legally valid in most states. If you choose this low-cost alternative, however, you should still have an attorney read it through.

Assign Durable Power of Attorney

The durable power of attorney is another legal document that assigns to a designated person the task of taking care of your financial and social responsibilities should you become incompetent to take care of your affairs. You will need a lawyer to draw this up—and, of course, you will need to obtain permission from the designated party ahead of time.

Consider a Living Will or Medical Durable Power of Attorney

A living will or medical durable power of attorney will allow you to dictate your wishes for how you should be treated when you are seriously ill.

You may use a living will to prescribe what may and may not be done to you in the last hours or days before your death. Called the Natural Death Act in some states, the living will can prevent doctors or hospitals from attempting heroic measures in case of an irreversible and clearly terminal illness. The vast majority of states permit these living wills, and most allow them to be made without the assistance of a lawyer. You can usually obtain a simple form to sign from your local hospital (see the social work department) or your doctor's office.

When you sign a medical durable power of attorney (in some states this does not require a lawyer), you designate a trusted person to make decisions concerning your medical care after you are no longer able to make those decisions for yourself. You may make this a very simple assignment of responsibility to cover any and all medical decisions, or you may specify medical situations in which this person may or may not decide.

The June 1990 Supreme Court ruling, *Cruzan v. Missouri*, illustrates the importance of both the living will and the medical durable power of attorney. The background to this ruling was a 1983 auto accident that left twenty-eight-year-old Nancy Cruzan in a persistent vegetative state. Ms. Cruzan remained in a coma for several years. In 1988 the Missouri State Supreme Court turned down the family's request to remove a feeding tube from their daughter's body. The family then appealed to the United States Supreme Court, which ruled in

June 1990 that the State of Missouri had a right to deny withdrawal of the feeding tube because there was a lack of "clear and convincing evidence" that this was what Nancy Cruzan would have wanted. The Supreme Court ruling will make it increasingly difficult in Missouri and possibly New York (where standards for evidence are stricter than in other states) to settle similar cases if there is no "clear and convincing evidence." Such evidence can be provided by a living will and a medical durable power of attorney.

If you live in Missouri or New York, therefore, and there is some question toward the end of your illness about how far to go in your treatment, only a living will and a medical durable power of attorney will ensure clarity and certainty. Their absence could spell confusion and heartache for your loved ones. In other states, stating your wishes to a family member is usually sufficient. Writing down your intentions, however, will remove any doubt and can relieve a relative forced to make a difficult decision of a burden of doubt and guilt.

Bill keeps copies of both of these documents outside his office for patients and passersby to read, take, and complete in the privacy of their homes. We would urge you to ask your doctor for such forms and then spend some time considering the possibilities and discussing them with your loved ones. Facing decisions about the end of life is not easy, but it can pay big benefits in terms of your family's peace and security.

Plan Your Estate

We don't have space in this book to provide details in this area, but suffice it to say that a carefully planned estate can be handed over more easily and rewardingly to heirs than one that is unplanned. By a few relatively simple maneuvers, you could save for your heirs thousands of dollars that otherwise would go for taxes.

Don't underestimate your assets. When you consider your liquid assets plus your home and land, you may exceed the federally determined maximum dollar amount that can be passed on to your family tax-free. We suggest that you contact a lawyer or financial planner for help.

Make Funeral Arrangements

You may find this topic too morbid to consider, especially if you've been told your chances for recovery are good. On the other hand, you may want to ensure that your wishes are carried out and spare your loved ones the burdens of planning and expense (which can be considerable) by looking into arrangements ahead of time. Most funeral directors are more than happy to discuss prepaid funerals or simply preplanned funerals. These are worth considering even if your death is still years down the road.

Get Your Paperwork in Order

Many families delegate certain tasks, such as keeping the checkbook and paying the bills, to one person. But pandemonium may break out if that person becomes gravely ill or dies without passing on what he or she knows. It is only considerate, therefore, to make sure that your bills, assets, and important papers are in order and easy to locate. Taking inventory of these papers could save your loved ones innumerable headaches. Papers to consider include wills, living wills, documents granting durable power of attorney and medical durable power of attorney, health insurance papers, disability policies, Veterans Administration papers, birth certificates, bank notes, stock certificates, safe deposit box keys, deeds of trust, mortgages, and notes bequeathing special items (such as antiques or fine jewelry) to loved ones.

What You Can Do: Personal and Spiritual Steps

Finally, in addition to taking practical steps to adjust to a life that has drastically changed, there is much you can do to explore and express your own attitudes and feelings. If you have been to the precipice and looked to the other side, your perspective has undoubtedly changed. You know that your life from here on out must be different. But how? What can you do to explore life after cancer? We suggest you try the following.

- Live one day at a time. Cherish each day for its individual blessings. Savor every pleasure. Express gratitude for the privilege of life and the gift of one more day. Thank God for the little blessings of the day.

- Ask for God's help to make it through the pressures and trials of that day. Don't worry how you will make it through the week or the month. Just take your troubles (and your joys) as they come.

- Don't be afraid of your thoughts or fears. Share them with God in prayer. Or share them with a friend or loved one. Or do both.

- Rearrange your priorities in life. Put people and relationships ahead of things and ambitions. Put God ahead of all.

- Don't be afraid to cry. Tears are a gift that help cleanse the soul and soothe the nerves.

- Laugh! Rent a funny video or read a funny book. Laughter is another gift that brings peace and rest to the soul. And there is some medical evidence that laughter can help heal the body as well.

- Scream when you have to. There are times when we feel angry at cancer or God or people—or just overcome with physical or emotional pain. At such times, it can be emotionally healthy to just let loose with a scream. While screaming at other people is not productive, just screaming (somewhere alone) can help us release that anger or frustration.

- Hug a child. Try to give love to others any opportunity that you can.

- Visit a forgotten friend and reminisce together over old pleasant memories.

- Visit a forgotten enemy. Try to pull down old walls and heal old wounds.

- Don't be afraid of your sexuality. Cancer need not limit your expression of sexual love to your mate. But if your condition or treatment does limit your sexual involvement, make loving touch an ongoing part of your relationship.

- Make a gift for an unborn grandchild. This will be one way for your life and love to pass down to another generation.

- Prepare an audiotape or video in which you describe the passions of your life—your loves, dreams, concerns for your family and the human race. Pass this on to your family or friends.

- Find a support group if sharing your burdens with others helps you.

- Make Jesus Christ a more prominent part of your day. Spend a quiet time once a day reading from the Bible and praying to God. Try to think of your prayer and Bible reading as a kind of dialogue with God: In Scripture, the Lord talks to you; in prayer you respond. Many cancer patients have found the Psalms to be especially moving and helpful.

- Keep your body as healthy as it can be, even with your illness. To the best of your ability, keep your weight stable, and try to keep up your strength. Eat nutritious food, and exercise as much as you can. All these efforts will help your body fight cancer and help you keep your spirits up as well.

- Men, grow a beard—or shave off the one you have. Women, try a new hairdo. Don't be afraid to try something different. If your hair is falling out in response to chemotherapy, invest in a really great wig.

- Put on your makeup. Buy a new outfit. Do whatever you can to present as good an appearance as possible.

- Be creative. Make something, write a song, or just rearrange your kitchen counters. Try to leave your mark on the world today by doing something to make it a fresher, more enjoyable place to be.

- Spend more time with your family—you never know how much time you have left with them. Don't keep putting off special, fun times. Consider each moment together as precious, an experience you may never enjoy again.

- Think of some other way to enjoy life more and make this world a better place.

- Subscribe to *Coping Magazine*. This is a quarterly news magazine for cancer patients and their families. See the appendix for information on how to subscribe.

Thank You, Cancer?

The great Russian novelist, Alexander Solzhenitsyn, spent eight years in the miserable work camps of the Soviet Gulag. After suffering horrible indignities in his eight years' imprisonment, Solzhenitsyn nevertheless looked back on those years and prayed, "Thank you, prison." He could say those words because it was in prison that Solzhenitsyn found his soul.

Cancer can do for you what the Gulag did for Solzhenitsyn. It is a disease that we would not wish on anyone. Yet countless thousands have used the experience of cancer as an opportunity to find and heal their souls. If you can learn from this book both what cancer is all about and how to find and strengthen your soul in the process, then, whether you survive cancer or not, you have truly conquered it.

Appendix

For Further Help

American Brain Tumor Association
3725 North Talman Avenue
Chicago, IL 60618
312-286-5571
800-886-2282

American Cancer Society
1599 Clifton Road, N.E.
Atlanta, GA 30329
404-320-3333
800-ACS-2345
www.cancer.org

American College of Surgeons (Commission on Cancer)
55 East Erie Street
Chicago, IL 60611
312-664-4050

Breast Cancer Information Clearinghouse
www.nysernet.org/bcic

Coping Magazine
Media America, Inc.
2019 North Carothers
Franklin, TN 37064
615-790-2400

International Myeloma Foundation
2120 Stanley Hills Drive
Los Angeles, CA 90046
800-452-CURE

Lawyer Referral Service
American Bar Association
1155 East 60th Street
Chicago, IL 60637
312-988-5000

Leukemia Society of America
600 Third Avenue
New York, NY 10016
212-573-8484

Look Good . . . Feel Better Program
800-558-5005

Mayo Health Oasis Cancer Resource Center (Mayo Clinic)
www.mayo.ivi.com/ivi/mayo/common/htm/canhpage.htm

Mediconsult.com (specializes in prostate cancer)
www.mediconsult.com

National Alliance of Breast Cancer Organizations (NABCO)
1180 Avenue of the Americas, 2nd Floor
New York, NY 10036
212-719-0154

National Cancer Institute—Cancer Information Service
Executive Plaza North, Room 239-C
Bethesda, MD 20892
800-4-CANCER
(Note: from the Hawaiian island of Oahu, call 808-524-1234; call
this number collect from other Hawaiian islands.)
www.icic.nci.nih.gov

National Coalition for Cancer Survivorship
1010 Wayne Avenue, 5th Floor
Silver Springs, MD 20910
301-585-2616

National Consumer Insurance
Help Line
800-942-4242

National Hospice Organization
1901 North Moore Street, Suite 901
Arlington, VA 22209
800-658-8898

National Institutes of Health
9000 Rockville Pike
Bethesda, MD 20892
301-496-4000

Oncolink (University of Pennsylvania School of Medicine)
oncolink.upenn.edu

Ronald McDonald House
500 North Michigan Avenue
Chicago, IL 60611

United Ostomy Association
36 Executive Park, Suite 120
Irvine, CA 92714
714-660-8624

Notes

Chapter 2

1. We must add that information is still coming out on radiation. Some articles in research journals are now arguing that there is little or no risk from radon exposure. The issue is obviously not settled yet; in the meantime, it is still advisable to check the radon level in your home.

Chapter 4

1. *Mayo Clinic Proceedings*, 72(1): 54–65.

2. According to 1997 estimates. All facts and figures on cancer are taken from the American Cancer Society, *Cancer Journal for Clinicians*, 47(1): 5–27, and 47(4): 239–42.

3. There are many other, rarer, types of skin cancer, such as Bowen's disease, Merkel's cell cancer, skin sarcomas, and sweat gland tumors. Unfortunately, we do not have space in this volume to devote attention to these.

4. *CA: A Journal for Clinicians*, 46(4): 195–98.

Chapter 8

1. Adapted from a story told in Ronni Sandroff, "Unproven Cancer Therapies: How to Steer Your Patients Away from Danger," *Oncology Times*, March 1991, 11.

2. Barrie R. Cassileth, "Unorthodox Cancer Medicine," *Cancer Investigation*, 4(6): 591.

3. Sandroff, "Unproven Cancer Therapies," 11.

4. Barrie R. Cassileth and Deborah Berlyne, "Counseling the Cancer Patient Who Wants to Try Unorthodox or Questionable Therapies," *Oncology*, April 1989, 29–33.

5. Cassileth and Berlyne, 29–33.

6. Cassileth, "Unorthodox Cancer Medicine," 4(6): 529.

7. Kenneth Hagin, quoted in D. R. McConnell, A *Different Gospel: A Historical and Biblical Analysis of the Modern Faith Movement* (Peabody, MA: Hendrickson, 1988), 152.

8. Hagin, quoted in McConnell, *Different Gospel*, 157.

9. Price, quoted in McConnell, *Different Gospel*, 152.

10. Price, quoted in McConnell, *Different Gospel*, 154.

11. Price, quoted in McConnell, *Different Gospel*, 154.

12. McConnell, *Different Gospel*, 81.

13. McConnell, *Different Gospel*, 169, note 58.

14. Romans 8:22–23.

15. Our coverage of the Simontons is derived primarily from Gregory A. Curt, "Unsound Methods of Cancer Treatment," *Principles and Practice of Oncology Updates*, 4(12): 7.

16. O. Carl Simonton and Stephanie Matthews-Simonton, *Getting Well Again: A Step-by-Step Self-Help Guide to Overcoming Cancer for Patients and Their Families* (New York: Bantam, 1980, original ed. 1970).

17. Bernie Siegel, *Love, Medicine and Miracles* (New York: Harper & Row, 1986).

18. Siegel, *Love, Medicine and Miracles*, 6, 4.

19. Siegel, *Love, Medicine and Miracles*, 3.

20. Proverbs 3:7–8.

21. The research in the next three paragraphs is documented in Curt, "Unsound Methods," 7.

22. Bill Moyers, *Healing and the Mind* (New York: Doubleday, 1993), 199.

23. Moyers, *Healing and the Mind*, 216–17.

24. Moyers, *Healing and the Mind*, 332.

25. Moyers, *Healing and the Mind*, 247.

26. Isaiah 14:13–15; Ezekiel 28:1–2; Acts 12:21–23.

27. Siegel, *Love, Medicine and Miracles*, 9.

28. Siegel, *Love, Medicine and Miracles*, 11.

29. Siegel, *Love, Medicine and Miracles*, 179.

30. Siegel, *Love, Medicine and Miracles*, 180.

31. Siegel, *Peace, Love & Healing—Bodymind Communication & the Path to Self-Healing: An Exploration* (New York: Walker and Co., 1990).

32. Sandroff, "Unproven Cancer Therapies," 43.

33. The material on laetrile, immunoaugmentative, and metabolic therapies was taken from Curt, "Unsound Methods," Cassileth and Berlyne, "Counseling the Cancer Patient," and Sandroff, "Unproven Cancer Therapies."

34. This list is taken in part from chapter 4 of Dr. David Sneed and Dr. Sharon Sneed, *The Hidden Agenda: A Critical View of Alternative Medical Therapies* (Nashville: Thomas Nelson, 1991). If you want more information on alternative therapies, we highly recommend this book.

Chapter 9

1. Harold Kushner, *When Bad Things Happen to Good People* (New York: Avon, 1981).

2. Isaiah 49:15, 66:13; Hosea 1–3, 11:1–4, 11:7–9.

3. Luke 15:11–32.

4. Deuteronomy 7:6–9; Romans 3:20–28.

5. Psalm 147:5.

6. 1 Chronicles 29:11; Isaiah 40:22–23; Psalms 22:8, 47:7–8.

7. Psalms 135:6–7.

8. Matthew 10:29–30.

9. Genesis 18:25; Psalms 96:13, 97:2.

10. Ezekiel 18:20.

11. On the other hand, Romans 5:12 suggests that we may have sinned in Adam. If that is the case, punishment of Adam's sin could be punishment of ours. And we are not punished by God for a sin that was exclusively Adam's.

12. John 12:31, 14:30 NASB.

13. Luke 13:16.

14. 2 Corinthians 12:7.

Chapter 10

1. John 5:14.

2. John 9:3 TEV.

3. Luke 13:1–5.

4. Deuteronomy 7:6–9; Ephesians 2:8–9; Romans 3:20–28, 9:6–24; John 3:17.

5. Job 1:9–11.

6. Job 2:3.

7. Job 1:8.

8. David Watson, *Fear No Evil: One Man Deals with Terminal Illness* (Wheaton, IL: Harold Shaw, 1984), 122.

9. Bo Neuhaus, *It's Okay, God, We Can Take It* (Austin, TX: Eakin, 1986), 100.

10. Neuhaus, *It's Okay*, 75.

11. C. S. Lewis, *A Grief Observed* (New York: Seabury, 1961), 42.

12. Philip Yancey makes this point in *Where Is God When It Hurts?* (Grand Rapids, MI: Zondervan, 1977).

13. C. S. Lewis, *The Problem of Pain* (New York: Macmillan, 1944), 81.

14. Sheldon Vanauken, *A Severe Mercy* (New York: Harper & Row, 1977), 216.

15. 1 Peter 1:5–7.

16. Watson, *Fear No Evil*, 130–31.

17. James 1:2–4.

18. Romans 5:3–5; Romans 8:28–29; Hebrews 2:9–11.

19. John Hick suggests this line of argument in *Evil and the God of Love* (Norfolk, England: Collins, 1968).

20. 2 Corinthians 10:10.

21. Galatians 4:15, 6:11.

22. 2 Corinthians 12: 1–10.

23. 2 Corinthians 12:9.

24. Ecclesiastes 3:2; Job 14:5 (see also Psalms 39:4); Psalms 139:16, 116:15.

25. 2 Corinthians 12:9–10.

Chapter 11

1. Job 42:3–6.

2. David Watson, *Fear No Evil: One Man Deals with Terminal Illness* (Wheaton, IL: Harold Shaw, 1984), 129.

3. Watson, *Fear No Evil*, 131–32.

4. Watson, *Fear No Evil*, 132.

5. Bo Neuhaus, *It's Okay, God, We Can Take It* (Austin, TX: Eakin, 1986), 113.

6. Watson, *Fear No Evil*, 133.

Chapter 12

1. Exodus 22:4.

2. Exodus 32–33.

3. James 5:16–17.

4. Dennis Prager and Joseph Telushkin, *The Nine Questions People Ask about Judaism* (New York: Simon & Schuster, 1981).

5. Exodus 33:18–23; Numbers 20:9–12; Deuteronomy 3.

6. John Claypool, *Tracks of a Fellow Struggler* (Waco, TX: Word, 1974), 73.

7. C. S. Lewis, *A Grief Observed* (New York: Seabury, 1961), 9.

8. Luci Shaw, *God in the Dark: Through Grief and Beyond* (Grand Rapids, MI: Zondervan, 1989), 240.

9. Lewis, *The Problem of Pain* (New York: Macmillan, 1944); *Grief Observed*, 31.

10. Shaw, *God in the Dark*, 250.

11. Lewis, *Grief Observed*, 55.

12. Lewis, *Grief Observed*, 56.

13. Psalms 13:1–2.

14. Lamentations 3:2–3, 7–8, emphasis added.

15. Lamentations 3:22–23, 31, 33.

16. Philip Yancey eloquently elaborates on this in his superb work, *Where Is God When It Hurts?* (Grand Rapids, MI: Zondervan, 1977).

17. Bo Neuhaus, *It's Okay, God, We Can Take It* (Austin, TX: Eakin, 1986), 17.

18. Yancey, *Where Is God?*, 183.

19. Isaiah 63:9.

20. Jeremiah 31:20.

21. Hosea 11:8.

22. John 11:35.

23. John 1:1.

24. Isaiah 53:3 KJV.

25. David Watson, *Fear No Evil: One Man Deals with Terminal Illness* (Wheaton, IL: Harold Shaw, 1984), 136.

26. Dorothy Sayers, quoted in Yancey, *Where Is God?*, 181.

27. Neuhaus, *It's Okay*, 103.

28. Neuhaus, *It's Okay*, 88–89.

29. Watson, *Fear No Evil*, 135.

30. This story is taken from Yancey, *Where Is God?*

31. Proverbs 17:22.

32. Lewis, *Problem of Pain*, viii.

33. Stanley Hauerwas, *Naming the Silences: God, Medicine, and the Problem of Suffering* (Grand Rapids, MI: Eerdmans, 1990), 151.

34. Job 2:13.

35. Ann Landers, column in *Roanoke Times & World News*, 18 January 1992. Permission granted by Ann Landers and Creators Syndicate.

Chapter 13

1. 2 Samuel 12:15–18.

2. John 5:1–9. John Wimber pointed this out in his *Power Healing* (San Francisco: Harper & Row, 1987).

3. Philippians 2:25–27.

4. 2 Timothy 4:20.

5. Acts 20:4.

6. 1 Timothy 5:23.

7. Romans 8:21; 1 Corinthians 15:53.

8. 2 Corinthians 5:8.

9. Werner Schaafs, *Theology, Physics and Miracles* (Washington, D.C.: Canon, 1974).

10. C. S. Lewis, *Miracles* (New York: Macmillan, 1947), from ch. 13, "On Probability."

11. See Acts 9:40–42, 20:7–12.

12. Matthew 14:14, emphasis added.

13. Matthew 20:29–34, emphasis added.

14. John 14:12.

15. Mark 16:18.

16. James 5:14–15.

17. Irenaeus, *Against Heresies*, book 2, chapter 32, no. 4.

18. Augustine, *City of God*, book 22, chapter 8.

19. Francis MacNutt, *Healing* (Notre Dame, IN: Ave Maria Press, 1974), 45–46.

20. Jack Grazier, *The Power Beyond: In Search of Miraculous Healing* (New York: Macmillan, 1989), 192–93.

21. Ecclesiasticus 38:1–15 NJB.

22. Roell's story is excerpted from Francis A. MacNutt, *The Power to Heal*, (Notre Dame, IN: Ave Maria Press © 1976), used with permission of the publisher.

23. Psalms 31:15, 56:3–4, 103:3, 107:20; Isaiah 53:5.

24. Matthew 9:6–7; Mark 1:41.

25. Matthew 8:14–15, 20:29–34; Luke 22:49–51,14:2–4,13:10–13, 8:49–56, 7:14–15.

26. John 9:6–7; Mark 8:23; Matthew 14:35–36, 9:20–22.

27. Acts 9:13; 1 Corinthians 16:1; 2 Corinthians 1:1.

28. 1 Corinthians 4:7; James 1:17; Ephesians 2:8-10; Romans 3:22-24; Jeremiah 17:9.

29. MacNutt, *Healing*, 172-73.

30. James 5:16.

31. Matthew 9:22; Luke 8:48, 17:19, 18:42; Acts 14:9-10, 3:16, emphasis added.

32. MacNutt, *Healing*, 147-48.

33. Emphasis added.

34. Wimber, *Power Healing*.

35. Hebrews 11:39.

36. Mark 8:22-25.

Chapter 14

1. *Compassion in Dying v. Washington*, 79 F3d 790 (9th Cir. 1996).

2. *Quill v. Vacco*, 80 F3d 716 (2d Cir. 1996).

3. E. Catherine Moroney, "Three Choices for Death," *America* (November 21, 1992), 402.

4. This last sentence is adapted from Vigen Guroian, *Life's Living toward Dying* (Grand Rapids, MI: Eerdmans, 1996), 14.

5. Ecclesiastes 3:2.

6. Unfortunately, the courts have not seen the difference between primary intent and secondary effect. See George J. Annas, "The Promised End—Constitutional Aspects of Physician-Assisted Suicide," *New England Journal of Medicine*, 335:9 (August 29, 1996), 683, and Kathleen M. Foley, "Competent Care for the Dying Instead of Physician-Assisted Suicide," *New England Journal of Medicine*, 336:1 (January 2, 1997), 54.

7. E. J. Emanuel, D. L. Fairclough, E. R. Daniels, and B. R. Clarridge, "Euthanasia and Physician-Assisted Suicide: Attitudes and Experiences of Oncology Patients, Oncologists, and the Public," *Lancet* (June 29,

1996), 1805–10; cited in Joan Klein, "At Life's End, Americans Divided Over Choices," *Oncology Times*, December 1996, 75.

8. A poll conducted for the American Medical Association in December 1996 concluded that most Americans would not want physician-assisted suicide if they clearly understood they had other choices such as hospice and palliative care. "AMA Poll: The More Patients Know, the Less They Want Suicide Aid," *American Medical News*, 40:2 (January 13, 1997), 2, 22.

9. Peter B. Terry, M.D., "Euthanasia and Assisted Suicide," *Mayo Clinic Proceedings*, 70 (1995), 189.

10. Quoted in David Schiedermayer, M.D., "Oregon and the Death of Dignity," *Christianity Today* (Feb. 6, 1995), 6.

11. Hebrews 12:7–12.

12. Romans 5:3–5.

13. Van der Maas, van Delden, Pijnenborg, Looman, "Euthanasia and Other Medical Decisions Concerning the End of Life," *Lancet*, 338 (1991), 669–74; cited in Terry, 190.

14. Orlowski, Smith, and van Zwienen, "Pediatric Euthanasia," *American Journal of Diseases of Children*, 146 (1992), 1440–46.

15. Poll cited, performed by the Dutch government, in "A Reason to Die: Euthanasia Comes to Washington State," *Crisis* (October 1991), 45.

16. Allen Verhey, "Choosing Death: The Ethics of Assisted Suicide," *Christian Century* (July 17–24, 1996), 719.

17. Romans 8:21 KJV.

18. Genesis 1:27.

19. Matthew 25: 35–40.

20. C. Everett Koop, M.D.; used with permission.

21. Walker Percy, *Signposts in a Strange Land* (New York: Farrar, Straus and Giroux, 1991), 350–51.

22. Robert Lifton, *The Nazi Doctors and the Nuremberg Code* (New York: Oxford University Press, 1995).

23. Walker Percy, *The Thanatos Syndrome* (New York: Farrar, Straus, Giroux, 1987), passim, but esp. 358–62.

24. See Matthew 12:22–32.

25. Job 2:1–6, 9.

26. Colossians 1:17; Hebrews 1:3.

27. Psalms 100:3.

Glossary

adjuvant therapy—literally, "auxiliary" therapy. Treatment whose object is to prevent or stop the spread of cancer to other parts of the body. Often used after removal of cancer from one part of the body. Usually consists of either chemotherapy or hormonal therapy, but can involve radiation therapy as well.

AIDS—Acquired Immune Deficiency Syndrome, an infectious disease that damages the immune system and is nearly always fatal. AIDS is not a cancer, but it may make the body more susceptible to certain cancers.

antibodies—proteins manufactured by the white blood cells that attack an unwanted substance in the body—a cell, a virus, or another antibody. See immune system.

antigen—a substance that can cause the white blood cells to produce antibodies. The presence of certain antigens can indicate the presence of cancer in the body. See immune system.

APR (abdominal-perineal resection)—the most common operation for rectal cancer. The rectum and muscles of the anal sphincter are removed; this procedure usually then necessitates a colostomy.

artery—a blood vessel that carries blood away from the heart.

benign—(of a tumor) noncancerous.

biopsy—the evaluation of a piece of tissue to see if it is malignant. The only certain way to diagnose cancer.

bone marrow—the soft tissue on the inside of most bones where blood is manufactured.

bone-marrow transplant—the application of lethal doses of chemotherapy, followed by the implantation of healthy marrow after the chemicals have left the body.

315

brachytherapy—the use of radioactive implants or pellets that deliver radiation at very close range—usually within a body cavity.

carcinogen—any substance that tends to produce a cancer when introduced into the body.

carcinoma—a particular kind of malignant tumor.

CAT scan (also called a CT scan)—computerized axial tomography, a very sophisticated form of X ray that enables the insides of the body to be viewed in three-dimensional form.

cell—the basic building block of living tissues. It is comprised of a nucleus (the "brain" of the cell), cytoplasm surrounding the nucleus, and a cell wall enveloping the cytoplasm.

cervix—see uterine cervix.

chemistries—measurement of important salts, minerals, and proteins contained in blood plasma (serum).

chemotherapy—the introduction of chemicals (drugs) into the body in an effort to eliminate cancer.

chromosome—the arrangement of thousands of genes on a strand of material in the nucleus of the cell.

clinical trial—an experimental treatment of cancer, usually developed at a university hospital, that tests new ideas in an attempt to find better treatments.

cobalt—a metallic element that can be modified to emit radiation and used to kill cancer cells. This is one form of radiation therapy.

colon—the segment of large intestine that connects the small intestine to the rectum.

colostomy—a procedure that redesigns the large intestine so that feces leave the body through a hole in the abdominal wall, to be caught in an adhesive plastic sac.

copayment—The portion of a doctor or hospital bill that the insurance won't pay and for which the patient is responsible, according to a prearranged contract. Usually the insurance pays 80 percent and the patient pays 20 percent.

DNA—deoxyribonucleic acid molecules. One of the nucleic acids, molecules that are arranged in particular ways in the nucleus of a cell to create a gene.

Duke's stages—a system used for denoting the stage of a colon or rectal cancer. It ranges from stage A (the earliest) to stage D (the most advanced).

durable power of attorney—a legal document that assigns to a specified person the task of taking care of a person's financial and social responsibilities when that person no longer can.

endoscopy—a method of looking inside an organ or cavity and performing procedures, such as a biopsy and minor surgery. It typically involves the use of a flexible lighted tube that goes inside the organ or cavity through an incision or body orifice. (See chapter 3 for a complete explanation.)

enzyme—a body protein that sets off certain biochemical reactions within the body.

EOB (explanation of benefit)—a statement from an insurance company telling what services have been rendered and what is covered under the benefits of an insurance plan.

erythrocytes—see red blood cells.

estrogen—a female hormone.

gene—a cluster of several thousand DNA molecules arranged in such a way on a chromosome (in the nucleus of a cell) that they convey a piece of information. These arrangements determine the body's identifying characteristics—everything from body size to hair color. Genes are responsible for heredity and carry information from old cells to new cells.

germ-cell tumor—a form of cancer usually found in the testicles or ovaries.

hemoglobin—a substance in red blood cells that carries oxygen throughout the body.

Hodgkin's disease—a kind of lymphoma that tends to be found in younger patients and is highly curable.

hormonal therapy—a form of treatment that prevents cancer cells from growing by taking advantage of the hormonal needs of these cells.

hormone—a body protein that controls the growth, development, and metabolism of other parts of the body. Insulin, for example, is a hormone that is made in the pancreas, but that circulates widely to control blood sugar.

hospice—a special health care program that provides a combination of medical, spiritual, and psychological care to patients and their families during a terminal illness. Hospice care is usually given in the home, but can also take place in a nursing home or hospital.

immune system—the mechanisms of the body that attack any substance or object in the body that appears to be foreign, such as viruses, transplanted organs, and malignant cells. The immune system performs many other functions as well.

infiltrating cancer—see invasive cancer.

in situ **cancer**—cancer that has not traveled beyond its site of origin—for example, a breast cancer that is still within the walls of a breast duct.

interferons—proteins that activate the immune system when an enemy is perceived by the body. Genetically engineered interferons have been used as "biological therapy" to fight some cancers (see chapter 5).

invasive cancer—cancer that has traveled beyond its site of origin. Also called infiltrating cancer.

laser—an acronym for "light amplification by stimulated emission of radiation." An intense light focused on a tiny area that can vaporize and cut tissue with very little damage to surrounding structures.

leukemia—cancer of the white blood cells.

leukocytes—see white blood cells.

living will—a written document, varying from region to region, in which you specify your wishes for the last days or hours before death.

lobectomy—partial removal of the lung; common way to treat non-small-cell carcinoma.

lumpectomy—breast-cancer surgery that removes only the tumor, leaving the rest of the breast intact.

lymphoma—cancer of the lymph system.

lymph system—a system of vessels in the body that carries immune cells and waste products. It can also be an avenue for the spread of cancer cells.

malignant—cancerous.

mammogram—an X-ray procedure that checks the breast for cancer.

mastectomy—surgery that removes the entire breast, usually as a treatment for cancer.

Medicaid—government health insurance for the poorest sector of our society.

medical durable power of attorney—similar to durable power of attorney, but applies only to medical decisions. The specified person makes decisions regarding your medical care when you are unable to make them for yourself.

Medicare—government health insurance for senior citizens (over sixty-five years of age), the disabled, and people needing permanent kidney dialysis.

metastasis—the spread of cancer from its site of origin to other parts of the body.

micrometastasis—literally, "small change." The spread of tiny cancer cells to other parts of the body. By definition, these cells are undetectable, but may "take root" and grow into detectable tumors.

MRI—magnetic resonance imaging, use of a giant magnet to make intricate pictures of the inside of the body by reorienting the body's atoms. Sometimes preferred over X rays because it does not use radiation.

myeloma—often called multiple myeloma. Cancer of bone-marrow plasma cells that is spread throughout the skeletal system.

nucleus—see cell.

non-small-cell carcinoma—any of four different kinds of lung cancer, whose pathology and treatment differ significantly from small-cell carcinoma. Usually treated by surgery.

oat-cell carcinoma—see small-cell carcinoma.

oncogene—a gene that, when deregulated, initiates cancerous growth in a cell.

oncologist—a physician whose specialty is cancer—either in surgery, radiation therapy, or internal medicine (chemotherapy).

oncology—the study and treatment of cancer.

Pap smear (Pap test)—named for the late Dr. Papanicolaou. Routine microscopic examination of cells from the uterine cervix (mouth of the womb) to check for cancerous change.

pathology—generally, the study of diseased tissue. In cancer cases it usually refers to the evaluation of cancer tissue under a microscope.

peritoneum—sac or membrane surrounding the abdominal organs.

plasma—the liquid part of the blood, yellow in color, that contains salts, minerals, and protein. Examination of the plasma helps the oncologist determine many things about the health of the body. Also called serum.

platelets—also called thrombocytes. One of the three types of cells in the blood (the other two are red blood cells and white blood cells). Platelets promote blood clotting.

prognosis—the attempt to predict the course of a disease in coming days and months. The answer to questions such as, "What are my chances, Doc?" and "How much time do I have?"

prosthesis—any artificial body part; for example, an artificial breast worn inside a mastectomy brassiere.

prostate cancer—common form of cancer found in the prostate gland, which encircles the male urethra and produces part of the seminal fluid.

proteins—a complex molecule that is a basic constituent of all living cells.

radiation therapy—the use of a beam of energy to kill cancer cells.

radon—a radioactive gas emitted by certain types of soil and rock and shown to be a carcinogen.

rectum—the segment of large intestine that connects the colon to the anus.

red blood cells—also called erythrocytes. One of three kinds of blood cells (the others are platelets and white blood cells). Red blood cells carry oxygen in their hemoglobin molecules.

relapse—in cancer care, the opposite of remission. The cancer has reappeared after a period of not being detected.

relative risk—a way of indicating how likely a person who has been exposed to a specific cancer-causing agent is to develop a cancer. Expressed as a number and computed by comparing the exposed person's risk to the risk incurred by someone not exposed to that factor.

remission—in cancer care, the word used for the state when a patient has no apparent traces of cancer remaining.

screening—the process of looking for any disease (including cancer) while it is still without symptoms and most curable.

serum—see plasma.

sigmoidoscopy—a method of looking into the lowest part of the intestine.

small-cell carcinoma—a type of lung cancer, also called oat-cell carcinoma, distinguished by the distinctive shape of its cells and usually treated with chemotherapy. See non-small-cell carcinoma.

staging—the process of determining how far a cancer has advanced. Tests involved in this process may include: blood test, radiographic study, biopsy, and endoscopy.

surgery—a medical procedure that usually involves opening the skin (with either a scalpel or a laser). Surgery may be used to detect cancer, treat it, or both, and may involve removal of an organ or other body part.

tamoxifen—a potent hormone useful in controlling the growth of breast cancer cells.

testosterone—a male hormone responsible for most of the physical characteristics of men. Lowering testosterone levels through hormone manipulation can slow the growth of prostate cancer and provide relief from painful symptoms.

thrombocytes—see platelets.

tumor—literally, "a swelling." Overgrowth of tissue that has a different structure from surrounding tissue. A tumor may be either benign (noncancerous) or malignant (cancerous).

tumor board—a panel of many different kinds of medical specialists who pool their expertise to determine how best to help a cancer patient.

tumor marker—proteins and other substances in the blood that indicate the presence of cancer cells somewhere else. (See chapter 3 for a list of significant tumor markers.)

ultrasound—a machine that uses sound waves to make pictures of the inside of the body.

uterine cervix—the mouth of the uterus (womb).

urologist—a physician specializing in diseases (benign and malignant) of the urinary tract, which includes the bladder, urethra, ureters, and kidneys.

vein—a blood vessel that carries blood toward the heart.

white blood cells—also called leukocytes. One of three kinds of blood cells (the others are platelets and red blood cells). Critical tools in the body's immune system, these cells fight infection.

X ray—a form of electromagnetic radiation capable of penetrating tissue. Focused through the body and onto film, X rays can cause a "picture" to be made of a part of the body.

Index

AFP (alpha feta protein), 31
AIDS (acquired immune deficiency
    syndrome), 18
Alcohol, 22, 24
Alkaline phosphatase, 32
Alternative cancer therapies,
    153–74
American Cancer Society, 28, 29
    Screening Guidelines, 29
Artery, 40
Asbestos, 22
Attitude, as cancer cause/cure,
    161–69, esp. 165–66
Augustine, 230–31

Barium X-rays, 36
Barth, Karl, 270
Benzopyrenes, 15
Berlyne, Deborah, 157
Bills for treatment. See Health
    insurance; Medical expenses
Biological therapies for cancer,
    122–25
    gene therapy, 124
    monoclonal antibodies, 123–24
Biopsy, 38–41
Bladder cancer, 16, 22
Bone marrow
    biopsy, 40
    transplants, 121–22
Bonhoeffer, Dietrich, 271
BRCA oncogenes, 19, 49–52
Breast cancer, 47–65

adjuvant therapy, 56–61
bone marrow transplantation,
    65, 121–22
causes, 22, 48
chemotherapy, 62, 64
clinical trials, 61–62
conservation surgery, 53–54
ductal, 47, 57
follow-up, 65
genetic factors, 19–21, 49–52
hormone receptors, 59, 62–63
hormone therapy, 59, 62–64
lobular, 47, 57
mammogram, 29, 37–38
mastectomy, 54–56
reconstructive surgery, 56
screening, 29
stages of, 27, 57–58
tamoxifen, 59, 62–64
treatment options, 60–65
Bronchoscopy, 42
Burton, Dr. Lawrence, 169–70

CA-125, 32
CA15–3, 32
CA19–9, 32
CA27.29, 32
Cancer
    American beliefs and, 157–58
    defined, 2
    educated Americans and,
        154–57
    faith healing, 158–61

immunoaugmentive therapy, 153–54, 169–70
metabolic therapies, 170–73
psychological therapy, 161–69
questions to ask, 173–74
unproven therapies, 153–74
See also entries by cancer type
Carcinogen, 15
Caregivers, 220–22, 289–91
Cassileth, Barrie, 154, 157
CAT scan (computerized axial tomography), 33–34, 38
CBC, 30
CEA, 31, 34
Cell, definition, 2
illustrated, 3
Centro Medico Del Mar, 173
Cervical cancer, 16, 22
Chemotherapy, 115–23
artificial veins, 121
bone marrow transplants, 121–22
drugs used, 116–18
effects, 115
in breast cancer, 62
myths, 116
side effects, 115–16, 118–121
Chromosomal overamplification, 9
Chromosome, 4–5
Clinical trials, 61–62
CML (chronic myelogenous leukemia), 8
Cobalt. See Radiation, in cancer treatment
Coffee enemas, 172
Colon and rectal cancer, 83–92
causes, 83–84
CEA, 31

diagnosis, 85–86
genetic factors, 19
numbers, 83
polyps, 85
stages, 88
surgery, 87–89
treatments, 88–92
Colonoscopy, 43–44
Colostomy, 87–88
Colposcopy, 44
Contreras, Dr. Ernesto, 173
Costs of treatment. See Health insurance; Medical expenses
Cousins, Norman, 220
CSF (colony-stimulating factors), 125
Curt, Gregory A., 154–55
Cystoscopy, 44

Detoxification, 172
Dietary fiber. See Fiber, dietary
DNA (deoxyribonucleic acid), 3
Down syndrome, 9
Ductal cancer. See Breast cancer, ductal
Duplication
cellular, 4–5
chromosomal, 9

East West Center for Macrobiotics, 171
EGD (Esophagogastroduodenoscopy), 42–43
Emotions, in cancer, 219–20
Endometrial cancer, 22
Endoscopy, 41–45
ERCP (endoscopicretrograde cholangiopancreatography), 43

Esophagus, cancer of, 16, 22, 44
Estrogens, as therapy, 22, 48
Evil, the problem of, 175–203
Expenses of treatment. See Health
    insurance; Medical expenses
Experimental/unapproved drugs,
    149–50

Faith healing, radical, 158–68
    denial of symptoms, 161
    theological flaws, 167–68
    See also Healing
Fiber, dietary, 16, 22, 24, 48
Forgiveness, 250–51, 287–88
Free will, 190–91
Freedom of choice, 266–68
Freeman, Hobart, 161

Gallbladder, cancer of, 22
Gene, 3–4, 7–9
Gene therapy, 124
Genetic factors in cancer, 19–20,
    49–52
Genetic testing, 50–52
Germ line, 49–50
God
    and chance 176–77
    and healing, 223–56
    and mystery, 199–203
    and punishment for sin, 178,
    182–83
    and Satan, 179
    and suicide, 265–66, 270,
    271–73
    arguing with, 205
    his love, 184
    his power, 177
    his silence, 208–13

his suffering, 213–17
    speaking through others, 218

Hagin, Kenneth, 159, 160, 161
Hair loss in chemotherapy, 118
Healing, 194–97, 223–56
Health insurance
    case manager, 149
    experimental/unapproved
    drugs, 149–50
    government plans, 140–44
    insurance problems, 147–50
    managed health care, 144–46
    paperwork, 146–47
    private, 139–40
    uninsured patient, 151–52
HMOs (health maintenance orga-
    nizations), 144–46
Hospice, 274–83
    history, 276
    benefits, 277–82
    restrictions, 282
Human chorionic gonadotropin
    (HCG, beta), 31

IEP (immunoelectrophoresis),
    31–32
Immune system, 17–18
Immunoaugmentative therapy,
    153–54, 169–70
in situ carcinoma
    ductal, 47
    lobular, 47
Insurance. See Health Insurance
Interferons, 125
Intraductal carcinoma. See in situ
Intralobular carcinoma. See in situ
Jaundice, 43

Jesus, 183, 192, 213–16, 224–25,
  228–29, 248–49, 250, 251, 254,
  265, 271, 272, 299
Job, 183, 185, 201, 206, 211, 212,
  221, 272

Kelly, Dr. William, 171
Kenyon, E.W., 159
Kevorkian, Dr. Jack, 258, 277–78
Koch, Dr. William, 170–71
Koop, Dr. Everett, 270
Kushi Foundation, 171
Kushner, Rabbi Harold, 176–77

Laetrile, 169
Laparoscopy, 44–45
Laser surgery, 111–12
LDH (lactate dehydrogenase), 31
Leukemia, chronic myelogenous
  (CML), 8, 122
Lewis, C.S., 187, 188, 209–11,
  212, 221, 228
Li-Fraumeni syndrome, 19
Life expectancy, in cancer. See
  entries by cancer type
Lifton, Robert, 271
Lobular carcinoma. See Breast
  cancer
Lung cancer
  causes, 16
  chemotherapy, 68–69
  non-small cell, 69–73
  prognosis, 68–69, 71–72
  small-cell, 67–69
  smoking and, 65–67, 73
  surgery, 69–71
  treatment options, 68–69
Lymph system, 40–41

nodes, 40–41
Lymphoma, 40–41

MacNutt, Francis, 231, 235, 241,
  250, 252, 253, 254
Mammogram, 29, 37–38
Managed health care, 144–46
Marrow, bone. See Bone marrow
Mastectomy, 54–56
McConnell, D.R., 161
McDermott, Joan, 245–48, 251,
  252, 253, 254
Mediastinoscopy, 44
Medicaid, 143–44
Medical expenses
  increased costs, 138
  payment strategies, 138–46
Medicare, 140–43
Megavitamin therapy, 171–73
Melanoma, 14, 16–17. See also
  Skin cancer
Metabolic therapies, 170–73
Mind over matter, 161–69
Miracles, 227–35, esp. 233
Monoclonal antibodies, 123–24
MRI (magnetic resonance imag-
  ing), 34–35
Multiple myeloma. See Myeloma,
  multiple
Myeloma, multiple, 27, 40, 47
Mystery, 199–203

Natural therapies. See Biological
  therapies for cancer
Negative confession, 159–60
Netherlands, physician-assisted
  suicide, 266
Neuhaus, Bo, 186, 202, 216–18, 220

Nieper, Hans, 173
Nuclear medicine, 36–37
Nucleic acids. See DNA
Nucleus, 3

Oat-cell carcinoma. See Small-cell
  carcinoma
Off label drugs, 150
Oncogene, 6–9, 13, 17–18, 19, 59
Orthomolecular treatment,
  171–73
Ovarian cancer, 31, 92–99
  causes, 93
  numbers, 92
  stages, 95–96
  surgery, 94–95
  survival, 98–99
  symptoms, 93–94
  tests, 93–94
  treatments, 96–98

P-53 (oncogene), 9, 19
Paget's disease, 47
Pain, in cancer, 135–36
Pancreas, cancer of, 16
Pap test, 29
Paul, thorn in the flesh, 194–97
Pepper, Claude, 154
Percy, Walker, 270–71
Peritoneal fluid, biopsy, 39
PET (positron emission tomogra-
  phy), 37
Physician-assisted suicide, 257–73
Platelets, 28, 30
Pleural fluid, biopsy, 39
Pollutants as cancer risk, 14–15,
  22
Ponder, Landy, 241–45, 251, 254

PPOs (preferred provider organizations), 144
Prayer
  and forgiveness, 250–51
  and unworthiness, 249
  for healing, 248–56
  of faith, 251–53
  soaking, 253–55
Price, Fred, 159–60, 161
Prostate cancer, 32, 73–83
  advanced cancer options, 81–83
  grade of tumor, 74–77
  impotence, 78, 79, 82
  numbers increase, 73
  screening, 73
  treatment, 77–80
PSA screening (for prostate cancer), 32, 73, 75
Psychological states, and cancer,
  165–66

Quack cures. See Cancer,
  unproven therapies

Radiation, in cancer treatment,
  112–13
  effects, 112–13
  side effects, 114–15
  types, 113–14
  See also entries by cancer type
Radiation, in environment, 13–14
Radiographic studies, 33–38
Radon, 14, 24
Rearrangement, gene, 7
Red blood cells, 28
Relative risk issues, 20–22
Remission, in cancer, 133
Resources, 292

Responsibilities, of cancer
  patients, 136
Rights of cancer patients, 129–36
  See also Treatment
RNA (ribonucleic acid), 7
Russell, Bertrand, 272

Saccharin, 22
Sandroff, Ronni, 169
Satan, 179
Schmidt, Roell, 235–40, 251, 253,
  254
Screening guidelines, 29
Shaw, Luci, 209–10, 212, 218
Siegel, Bernie, 161, 163–69
Silicone breast implant, 22
Simonton, O. Carl and Stephanie
  Matthews, 161–63
Skin cancer
  causes, 101–2
  increased risk, 100
  risk factors, 102–3
  stages, 105
  surgery, 105–6
  survival, 101, 105
  treatment, 107–8
  types, 100, 104
Small-cell carcinoma (lung can-
  cer), 67–69
Smoking, and lung cancer, 65–67,
  73
Solzhenitsyn, Alexander, 300
Spinal fluid, biopsy, 39–40
Staging, of cancer, 26–45
Stent, 43
Suffering, 161, 175–203, 257–73
  in cancer, 135–36

Suicide. See Physician-assisted
  suicide
Sunlight, 13–14, 16–17, 24
Suppressor gene, 8–9
Surgery in cancer treatment,
  110–11
  laser surgery, 111–12
  myths, 111
  when used, 110–11

Tada, Joni Eareckson, 202
Therapy. See Alternative cancer
  therapies; entries by cancer type
Throat cancer, 16
Tobacco. See Lung cancer, smoking and
Translocation, 7
Treatment
  discontinuing, 133
  questions to ask, 126–27,
  131–32
  second opinion, 133–34
  side effects, 132
Tumor board, 125–26
Tumor markers, 30–32
TURP (transurethral resection of
  the prostate), 77–78

Ultrasound, 36
Uninsured patient, 151–52
Uterine cancer. See Cervical
  cancer; Endometrial cancer

Vagina, cancer of, 17
Vanauken, Sheldon, 188
Vein, 28, 41
Venipuncture, 28, 29

Verhey, Allen, 268
Virus, 7, 13
Vitamin deficiency, 18
Vitamins, 24, 171–72

Watson, David, 186, 187, 202,
    220, 221, 253

White blood cells, 28, 30
Wills, 294–96
Wolterstorff, Nicholas, 221
Wurmbrand, Richard, 218

X-rays, 14, 33, 36, 43